Retinal Detachment

Colour Manuals in Ophthalmology

Contact Lenses in Ophthalmology
by Michael Wilson and Elisabeth Millis

Glaucoma
by Jack J. Kanski and James A. McAllister

The Eye in Systemic Disease
by Jack J. Kanski and Dafydd J. Thomas

Uveitis
by Jack J. Kanski

Vascular Disorders of the Ocular Fundus
by R.H.B. Grey

Retinal Detachment

A Colour Manual of Diagnosis and Treatment

Second edition

Jack J. Kanski, MD, MS, FRCS, FRCOphth

Consultant Ophthalmic Surgeon,
Prince Charles Eye Unit,
King Edward VII Hospital, Windsor

Zdenek J. Gregor, FRCS, FRCOphth

Consultant Ophthalmic Surgeon,
Moorfields Eye Hospital, London

Artwork by T.R. Tarrant

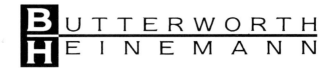

BUTTERWORTH
HEINEMANN

Butterworth-Heineman Ltd
Linacre House, Jordan Hill, Oxford OX2 8DP

 A member of the Reed Elsevier plc group

OXFORD LONDON BOSTON
MUNICH NEW DELHI SINGAPORE SYDNEY
TOKYO TORONTO WELLINGTON

First published 1986
Second edition 1994

British Library Cataloguing in Publication Data
Kanski, Jack J.
  Retinal Detachment: Colour Manual of
  Diagnosis and Treatment. – 2Rev.ed. –
  (Colour Manuals in Ophthalmology)
  I. Title II. Gregor, Zdenek III. Series
  617.73

ISBN 0 7506 1768 3

Library of Congress Cataloguing in Publication Data
Kanski, Jack J.
  Retinal detachment : a colour manual of diagnosis and treatment/
  Jack J. Kanski, Zdenek J. Gregor; artwork by T.R. Tarrant. – 2nd ed.
  p. cm. – (Colour manuals in ophthalmology)
  Includes bibliographical references and index.
  ISBN 0 7506 1768 3
  1. Retinal detachment – Handbooks, manuals, etc. I. Gregor,
  Zdenek J. II. Title. III. Series.
  [DNLM: 1. Retinal Detachment – diagnosis. 2. Retinal Detachment
  – therapy. WW 270 K16r]
  RE603.K35   94–27820
  617.7'3–dc20   CIP

Composition by Scribe Design, Gillingham, Kent
Printed by Cambus Litho, East Kilbride

Contents

Preface

The primary aim of this book is to give the trainee ophthalmol-ogist a systematic overview of the diagnosis and management of the various types of retinal detachment. Because many advances in vitreoretinal surgery have taken place since the first edition was published nine years ago, it has been necessary to completely revise the second edition and add a considerable amount of new material, particularly in the treatment of complex retinal detachments by vitrectomy. Many new illustrations have also been added and the number of chapters increased from ten to twelve. We are extremely grateful to Terry Tarrant for the superb artwork.

J.J.K.
Z.J.G.

1 Introduction

Definitions and classifications

Vitreoretinal traction

Vitreoretinal traction is a force exerted on the retina by structures originating in the vitreous. The two main types are (a) **dynamic** and (b) **static**. The difference between the two is crucial in understanding the pathogenesis of the various types of retinal detachment (RD).

Dynamic vitreoretinal traction

Dynamic traction is induced by rapid eye movements and exerts a centripetal force towards the vitreous cavity. It plays an important role in the pathogenesis of retinal tears and rhegmatogenous RD (see Figure 3.1).

Static vitreoretinal traction

Static traction is independent of ocular movements. It plays an important role in the pathogenesis of tractional RD and proliferative vitreoretinopathy. The following are the three main types:

1. **Tangential** (surface) traction which acts parallel to the surface of the retina as a result of contraction of epiretinal or subretinal membranes (see Figure 3.16).
2. **Anteroposterior** traction in which the pull is from the retina posteriorly to the vitreous base (see Figure 3.17).
3. **Bridging** (trampoline) traction in which the pull is from one part of the retina to another, usually along the detached posterior hyaloid surface (see Figure 3.18).

Retinal breaks

A retinal break is a full-thickness defect or discontinuity in the sensory retina. Breaks can be classified according to (a) **pathogenesis**, (b) **morphology** and (c) **location**.

Pathogenesis

Retinal breaks are of the following two types:

1. **Tears** are primarily caused by dynamic vitreoretinal traction. They have a predilection for the upper fundus (temporal more than nasal).
2. **Holes** are primarily caused by chronic atrophy of the sensory retina. They have a predilection for the temporal fundus (upper more than lower) and are less dangerous than tears.

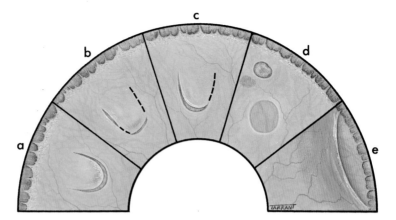

Figure 1.1 Retinal tears: (*a*) complete U-tear; (*b*) linear tears; (*c*) L-shaped tear; (*d*) operculated tear; (*e*) dialysis

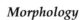

Morphology

Retinal holes are round or oval. Retinal tears can have one of the following five configurations:

1. **U-tears**, also described as horseshoe or flap tears, consist of a flap which is attached to the retina at its base and two posterior extensions (horns) which meet at the apex (Figure 1.1*a*). The vitreous gel is attached to the flap of the tear and the arrow of the tear always points posteriorly.
2. **Incomplete U-tears**, which can be linear (Figure 1.1*b*), L-shaped (Figure 1.1*c*) or J-shaped, are often paravascular.
3. **Operculated tears** in which the flap is completely torn away from the retina by detached vitreous gel (Figure 1.1*d*).
4. **Dialyses** are circumferential tears along the ora serrata (Figure 1.1*e*) so that vitreous gel is attached to their posterior margins.
5. **Giant tears** involve 90° or more of the circumference of the globe (see Figure 3.11, *bottom*). They are a variant of U-shaped tears with the vitreous gel attached to the anterior margin of the break. Giant tears are most frequently located in the immediate post-oral retina or less commonly the equator.

Location

1. **Oral** breaks are located within the vitreous base.
2. **Post-oral** breaks are located between the posterior border of the vitreous base and equator.
3. **Equatorial** breaks are near the equator.
4. **Postequatorial** breaks are behind the equator.
5. **Macular** breaks (invariably holes) are at the fovea.

Retinal detachment

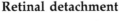

The following three forces promote attachment of the normal sensory retina to the underlying retinal pigment epithelium (RPE):

Introduction

1. The RPE pump which creates a negative pressure in the subretinal space.
2. Intercellular mucopolysaccharide matrix between the sensory retina and RPE.
3. Interdigitation of the RPE cell processes with the rods and cones.

RD is caused by a breakdown of these forces resulting in separation of the sensory retina from the RPE by subretinal fluid (SRF). The two main types are (a) **rhegmatogenous** and (b) **non-rhegmatogenous**.

Rhegmatogenous RD

Rhegmatogenous RD is caused by a retinal break which permits SRF derived from synchytic (liquefied) vitreous to gain access to the subretinal space. The aim of treatment of rhegmatogenous RDs is closure of the causative break, usually by scleral buckling.

Non-rhegmatogenous RD

Non-rhegmatogenous RD is not caused by a retinal break. The following are the two main types:

1. **Tractional** in which the sensory retina is pulled away from the RPE by contracting vitreoretinal membranes; the source of SRF is unknown.
2. **Exudative** (serous, secondary) in which SRF derived from the choroid gains access to the subretinal space through damaged RPE.

Posterior vitreous detachment

Posterior vitreous detachment (PVD) is a separation of the cortical vitreous from the internal limiting membrane (ILM) of the sensory retina posterior to the vitreous base. PVD can be classified according to the following characteristics:

1. **Onset** into the following two types:
   (a) *Acute* develops suddenly and may be complete soon after onset.
   (b) *Chronic* develops gradually and may take weeks or months to become complete.
2. **Completeness** into the following two types:
   (a) *Complete* in which the entire vitreous cortex detaches up to the posterior margin of the vitreous base.
   (b) *Incomplete* in which residual vitreoretinal attachments remain.
3. **Presence of a defect in the posterior vitreous surface** into the following two types:
   (a) *Rhegmatogenous* in which a defect is present.
   (b) *Non-rhegmatogenous* in which a defect is absent.

Introduction

Rhegmatogenous RD is associated with acute rhegmatogenous PVD; tractional RD is typically associated with chronic, incomplete, non-rhegmatogenous PVD; and exudative RD is usually unassociated with PVD.

Applied anatomy

Ora serrata

The ora serrata is the junction between the retina and ciliary body (Figure 1.2). The nasal ora is characterized by tooth-like extensions of retina onto the pars plana (dentate processes) which are separated by oral bays. In the temporal ora the dentate processes are blunt or absent. Clinically insignificant congenital lesions are small glistening 'oral pearls'. In the phakic eye the

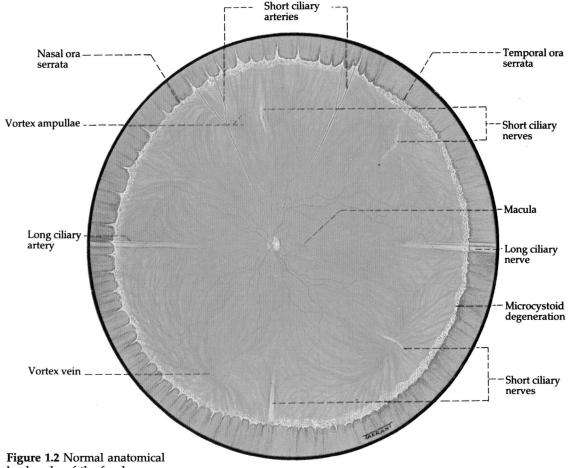

Figure 1.2 Normal anatomical landmarks of the fundus

5

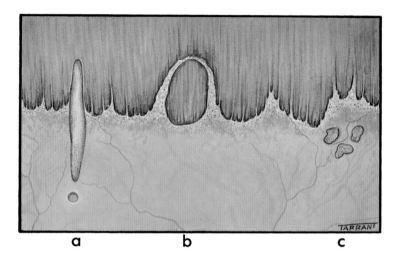

a   b   c

Figure 1.3 Normal variants of the ora serrata; (*a*) meridional fold with a small hole at its base; (*b*) enclosed oral bay; (*c*) granular tissue

ora cannot be visualized without scleral indentation whereas in the aphakic eye visualization is possible without indentation, provided the pupil is large. Externally the ora corresponds to the insertions of the rectus muscles. In the emmetropic eye this is located 7 mm behind the limbus temporally and 6 mm nasally. At the ora, the sensory retina is fused with the RPE and choroid. This adhesion, which is weaker nasally than temporally, acts as a barrier to the spread of SRF into the pars plana. However, there is no equivalent adhesion between the choroid and sclera, so that choroidal detachments invariably progress anteriorly to involve the ciliary body. The following congenital anomalies may occasionally have clinical significance (Figure 1.3):

1. **A meridional fold** is a small radial fold of retina in line with a dentate process which may occasionally have a small retinal hole at its base (Figure 1.3*a*).
2. **An enclosed oral bay** is a small island of pars plana surrounded by retina as a result of meeting of two adjacent dentate processes (Figure 1.3*b*). It should not be mistaken for a retinal hole because it is located anterior to the ora serrata.
3. **Granular tissue** characterized by multiple, tiny, white opacities within the vitreous base can sometimes be mistaken for very small peripheral opercula (Figure 1.3*c*).

Pars plana

The ciliary body starts 1 mm from the limbus and extends posteriorly for about 6 mm. The first 2 mm consist of the pars plicata and the remaining 4 mm consist of the flattened pars plana. Clinically insignificant congenital anomalies are transparent cysts located between the non-pigmented and the pigmented ciliary epithelium (pars plana cysts). In order not to endanger the lens or retina, the ideal location for surgical incisions is 3 mm from the limbus in aphakic or pseudophakic eyes and 3.5 mm in phakic eyes.

Vitreous base

The vitreous base is a 3–4 mm wide zone that straddles the ora serrata (Figure 1.4). The collagen fibres of the vitreous are exceptionally dense and strongly adherent to the posterior pars plana and perioral retina. An incision through the mid-part of the pars plana will usually be located anterior to the vitreous base. If blunt-ended instruments are introduced into the eye through the vitreous base they may exert traction and give rise to a peripheral retinal tear. Because of the strong adhesion of the cortical vitreous at the vitreous base, following an acute PVD the posterior hyaloid surface remains attached to the posterior border of the vitreous base and any pre-existing perioral retinal holes within the vitreous base do not lead to RD. Severe blunt ocular trauma may cause an avulsion of the vitreous base with tearing of the non-pigmented epithelium of the pars plana along its anterior border and of the retina along its posterior border. Posterior tongue-like extensions and isolated islands of dense cortical vitreous associated with abnormally strong vitreoretinal adhesions may be the sites of retinal tears in eyes with acute PVD.

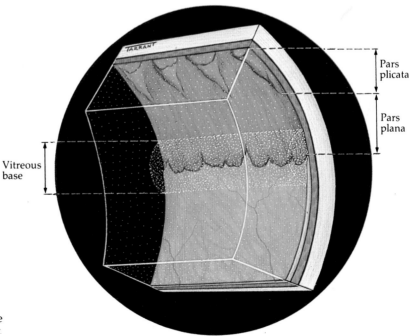

Figure 1.4 Anatomy of the vitreous base

Vitreoretinal adhesions

Normal adhesions

In the normal eye the peripheral cortical vitreous is loosely attached to the ILM of the sensory retina. Stronger attachments occur at the following sites:

1. Vitreous base – very strong.
2. Around the optic disc margin – fairly strong.
3. Around the fovea – fairly weak.
4. Peripheral retinal blood vessels – usually weak.

Abnormal adhesions

Occasionally, the following abnormally strong vitreoretinal adhesions are associated with retinal tear formation caused by dynamic vitreoretinal traction in eyes with acute PVD (see Chapter 3).

1. Posterior border of lattice degeneration.
2. Congenital cystic retinal tufts which are white, ovoid, inward projections of sensory retina located in the postbasal area.
3. Retinal pigment clumps.
4. Peripheral paravascular condensations.
5. Vitreous base anomalies such as posterior tongue-like extensions and isolated islands.
6. Areas of 'white-without-pressure'.

Long posterior ciliary arteries

The long posterior ciliary arteries accompanied by nerves are recognized as yellow lines that start behind the equator and run anteriorly in the 3 and 9 o'clock meridia. They divide the fundus into upper and lower zones (see Figure 1.2). The arteries run in the suprachoroidal space in line with the horizontal recti. Care should be taken not to damage them when draining SRF or performing intravitreal injections. Because these arteries supply the anterior uvea, obstruction to blood flow by a tight encircling band may result in anterior segment ischaemia. The short posterior ciliary arteries are not accompanied by nerves and may be difficult to identify ophthalmoscopically. The short ciliary nerves appear as peripheral yellow lines.

Vortex veins

The vortex ampullae are located just posterior to the equator in the 1, 5, 7, and 11 o'clock meridia (see Figure 1.2). Externally the vortex veins emerge from their scleral canals at variable distances from the equator. Frequently more than four vortex veins are present, and great care should be taken not to damage them when inserting a squint hook under the rectus muscles. The inferior vortex veins are at particular risk because they are usually located more anteriorly than the superior. Because the venous drainage of the anterior uvea is mainly via the vortex system, occlusion of the veins by a posteriorly placed tight encircling strap will cause congestion of the anterior segment. The vortex veins limit posterior extension of a choroidal detachment as they pass through the suprachoroidal space into their scleral canals.

Further reading

Foos, R. Y. (1974) Vitreous base, retinal tufts, and retinal tears. In *Retina Congress*, edited by C. D. J. Regan, pp. 259–280. New York: Appleton-Century-Crofts

Grignolo, A., Schepens, C. L. and Health, P. (1957) Cysts of the pars plana ciliaris. Ophthalmoscopic appearance and pathological description. *Archives of Ophthalmology*, **58**, 530–543

Lonn, L. I. and Smith, T. R. (1967) Ora serrata pearls. *Archives of Ophthalmology*, **77**, 809–813

Sigelman, J. (1980) Vitreous base classification of retinal tears: clinical application. *Survey of Ophthalmology*, **25**, 59–70

Spencer, L. M. and Foos, R. Y. (1970) Paravascular vitreoretinal attachments. *Archives of Ophthalmology*, **84**, 557–564

Spencer, L. M., Foos, R. Y. and Straatsma, B. R. (1970) Enclosed bays of the ora serrata. *Archives of Ophthalmology*, **83**, 420–425

Spencer, L. M., Foos, R. Y. and Straatsma, B. R. (1970) Meridional folds, meridional complexes and associated abnormalities of the peripheral retina. *American Journal of Ophthalmology*, **70**, 697–714

Straatsma B. R., Landers, M. B. and Kreiger, A. E. (1968) The ora serrata in the adult human eye. *Archives of Ophthalmology*, **80**, 3–20

2   Examination techniques

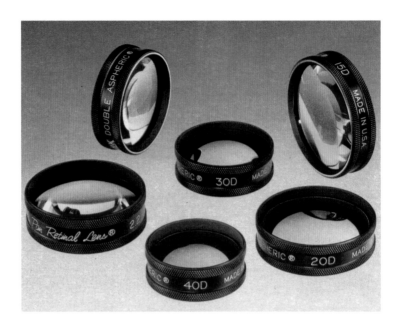

Figure 2.1 Condensing lenses used for indirect ophthalmoscopy

Standard indirect ophthalmoscopy

Condensing lenses

Condensing lenses of various powers and diameters are available for indirect ophthalmoscopy (Figure 2.1). The higher the power, the less the magnification, the shorter the working distance but the greater the field of view. The following lenses are currently available:

1. 15D (magnifies ×4; field about 40°) is good for examination of the posterior pole.
2. 20D (magnifies ×3; field about 45°) is the most commonly used for general examination of the fundus.
3. 25D (magnifies ×2.5; field about 50°).
4. 30D (magnifies ×2; field of 60°) has a shorter working distance and is useful when examining patients with small pupils.
5. 40D (magnifies ×1; field about 65°) is used mainly to examine small children.
6. Pan Retinal 2.2 (magnifies ×3; field about 55°).

Technique

1. Dilate both pupils well with 1% tropicamide and, if necessary, phenylephrine (2.5%, 5% or 10%) so that they will not constrict when exposed to a bright light.

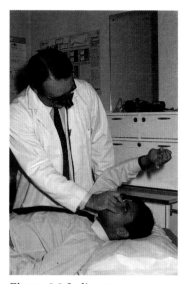

Figure 2.2 Indirect ophthalmoscopy – correct position

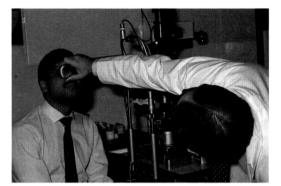

Figure 2.3 Indirect ophthalmoscopy – incorrect position

2. The patient should be in the supine position, with one pillow, on a bed, reclining chair or couch (Figure 2.2) and not sitting upright in a chair (Figure 2.3).
3. Darken the examination room.
4. Check the indirect ophthalmoscope for correct interpupillary distance and align the beam so that it is located in the centre of the viewing frame.
5. Instruct the patient to keep both eyes open at all times.
6. Take the lens into one hand with the flat surface facing the patient and at all times try to keep it parallel to the patient's iris plane.
7. If necessary, gently separate the patient's eyelids with the fingers.
8. Find the red reflex but do not turn the power of the light beam to maximum.
9. In order to enable the patient to get used to the light ask him to look up and then examine the superior peripheral fundus first.

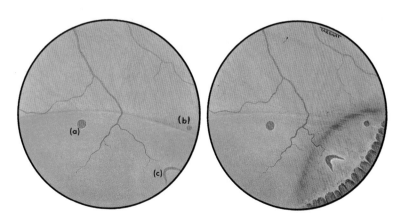

Figure 2.4 *Left*: appearance of retinal breaks without scleral indentation; *right*: with scleral indentation

10. Avoid the tendency to move towards the patient if you are having difficulty in seeing the fundus.
11. Be prepared to move around the patient and stand opposite the clock hour position to be examined. For example, when viewing the 9 o'clock meridian stand on the patient's left-hand side.
12. Ask the patient to move the eyes and head into optimal positions for examination. For example, when examining the extreme retinal periphery, ask the patient to look away from you.

Scleral indentation

Purpose

Scleral indentation should be attempted only after the art of indirect ophthalmoscopy has been mastered. Its main purpose is to enhance visualization of the peripheral retina anterior to the equator and to perform a kinetic evaluation of the retina. For example, Figure 2.4, *left*, shows a retinal hole (**a**) near the equator which can be seen without scleral indentation because the underlying choroid provides good contrast and the hole appears red. However, a small round hole (**b**) near the ora serrata or a small U-tear (**c**) near the posterior border of the vitreous base may be overlooked without scleral indentation. Figure 2.4, *right*, shows that with scleral indentation the small hole (**b**) is seen more easily because the contrast between the choroid and sensory retina is enhanced. Indentation also brings the peripheral fundus into view and enables the flap of the small U-tear (**c**) to be seen in profile. It should, however, be pointed out that scleral indentation may be hazardous in eyes with angle-supported anterior chamber intraocular lens implants or within a few weeks of cataract extraction where the incision has not completely healed.

Technique

1. Take the indentor into one hand; it can be either a specially designed T-shaped bar on a thimble or a simple unfolded paper clip.
2. To view the ora serrata at 12 o'clock, first ask the patient to look down and then apply the scleral indentor to the outside of the upper eyelid at the margin of the tarsal plate (Figure 2.5).
2. With the indentor in place, ask the patient to look up; at the same time advance the indentor into the anterior orbit parallel with the globe (Figure 2.6).
3. Align your eyes with the condensing lens and indentor and then exert gentle pressure and observe the mound created

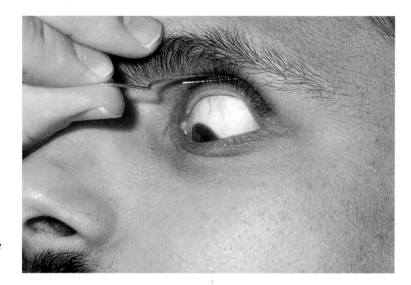

Figure 2.5 Insertion of a simple unfolded paper clip for scleral indentation

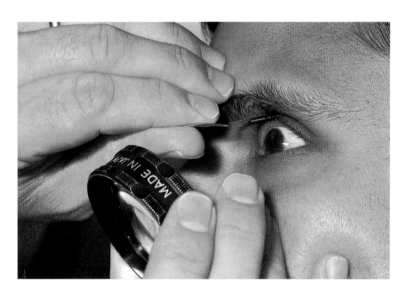

Figure 2.6 Scleral indentation

by the indentation in the fundus. At all times keep the indentor tangential to the globe because you will cause pain if indentation is perpendicular.

4. Move the indentor to an adjacent part of the fundus, making sure that your eyes, the condensing lens, the fundus image and the indentor are all in a straight line.

5. The entire fundus can usually be examined while indenting through the eyelids. Occasionally, in patients with very tight eyelids, indentation directly over the conjunctiva may be necessary in the 3 and 9 o'clock positions. If this is done gently, a topical anaesthetic may not be required.

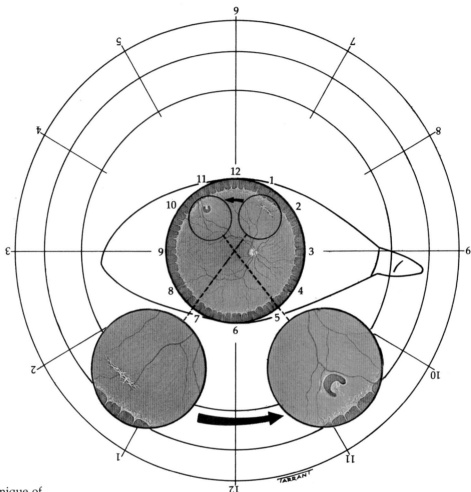

Figure 2.7 Technique of
drawing retinal lesions as seen
by indirect ophthalmoscopy

Fundus drawing

Technique

The image seen with the indirect ophthalmoscope is vertically
inverted and laterally reversed. This phenomenon can be used
to good advantage when drawing the fundus if the top of the
chart is placed towards the patient's feet (upside down). In this
way the inverted position of the chart in relation to the patient's
eye corresponds to the image of the fundus obtained by the
observer. For example, a U-tear at 11 o'clock in the patient's right
eye will correspond to the 11 o'clock position on the chart
(Figure 2.7). The same applies to the area of lattice degeneration
between 1 o'clock and 2 o'clock.

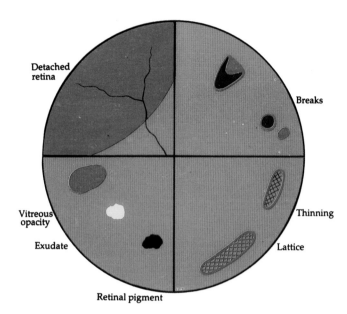

Figure 2.8 Colour code for retinal drawing

Colour code

Have available coloured pencils (red, blue, yellow, black, green) (Figure 2.8).

1. Record the boundaries of the RD by starting at the optic nerve and then extending to the periphery.
2. Draw detached retina in blue and flat retina in red.
3. Indicate the course of retinal veins with blue. Retinal arterioles are not usually drawn unless they serve as a special guide to an important lesion.
4. Draw retinal breaks in red with blue outlines; the flap of a retinal tear is also drawn in blue.
5. Thin retina is indicated by red hatchings outlined in blue; lattice degeneration is shown as blue hatchings outlined in blue; retinal pigment is black; retinal exudates yellow; and vitreous opacities green.

Slitlamp biomicroscopy

Purpose

Slitlamp biomicroscopy should be performed after the fundus has been drawn. The particular advantages are as follows.

1. The magnification of the slitlamp is useful in detecting small peripheral retinal breaks, especially in eyes with choroidal

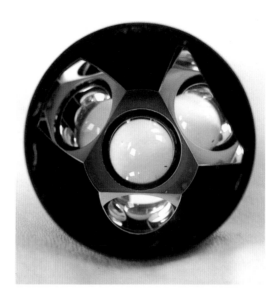

Figure 2.9 Goldmann triple mirror

atrophy in which the colour contrast between the choroid and sensory retina is reduced. It is also useful in deciding whether or not an area of very thin retina (as in lattice degeneration) contains small retinal holes.
2. Evaluation of the vitreous with respect to the presence of transvitreal membranes, vitreous opacities and PVD.
3. Evaluation of lesions at the posterior pole such as possible macular holes with high magnification.

The two main techniques for slitlamp examination of the fundus are: (a) **Goldmann triple-mirror** and (b) **biomicroscopic indirect ophthalmoscopy**.

Goldmann triple-mirror examination

The Goldmann triple-mirror contact lens consists of four parts; a central part and three mirrors set at different angles (Figure 2.9). It is important to be familiar with each part of the lens as follows:

1. **The central** part provides a 30° view of the posterior pole.
2. **The equatorial mirror** (largest and oblong shaped) enables visualization from 30° to the equator.
3. **The peripheral mirror** (intermediate in size and square shaped) enables visualization between the equator and the ora serrata.
4. **The gonioscopic mirror** (smallest and dome shaped) may be used for visualizing the extreme retinal periphery and pars plana. It is therefore apparent that the smaller the mirror the more peripheral the view.

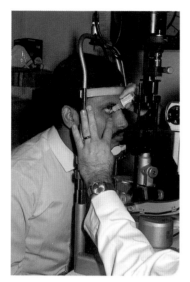

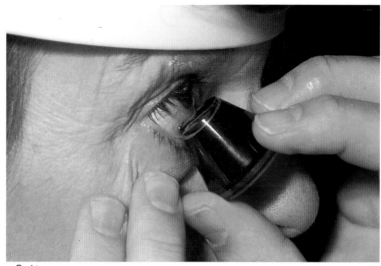

Figure 2.10 Instillation of topical anaesthetic

Figure 2.11 Insertion of triple mirror into lower fornix with patient looking up

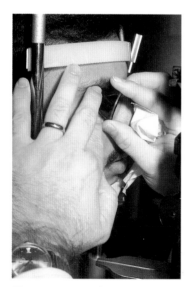

Figure 2.12 Triple mirror in position

Preliminary steps

1. Dilate the pupils as for indirect ophthalmoscopy.
2. Ask the patient to keep both eyes open at all times and not to move the head backward when the lens is being inserted.
3. Make sure that you have at hand high viscosity methylcellulose (or equivalent) to use as coupling fluid and soft tissues for cleaning the lens prior to insertion and for wiping excess coupling fluid from the patient's cheek.
4. Instil topical anaesthetic drops (Figure 2.10).
5. Insert coupling fluid into the cup of the contact lens but do not overfill; it should be no more than half full.
6. Ask the patient to look up, insert the inferior rim of the lens into the lower fornix (Figure 2.11) and press it quickly against the cornea so that the coupling fluid has no time to escape (Figure 2.12).
7. Ask the patient to look straight ahead and wipe away any excess coupling fluid (Figure 2.13).

When viewing with the triple mirror the image is upside down. This means that when you wish to view the 12 o'clock position in the peripheral fundus, you should position the mirror at 6 o'clock. The image in the mirror will not be laterally reversed as with indirect ophthalmoscopy so that lesions located to the left of 12 o'clock in the retina will also appear in the mirror on the left-hand side (Figure 2.14).

19

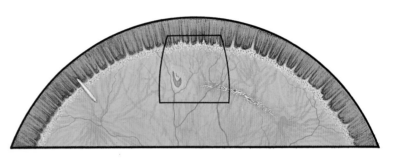

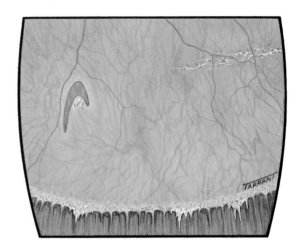

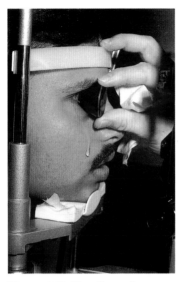

Figure 2.13 Overflow of coupling fluid onto the cheek

Figure 2.14 *Top*: U-tear left of 12 o'clock and an island of lattice degeneration right of 12 o'clock; *bottom*: the same lesions as seen with the triple mirror positioned at 6 o'clock

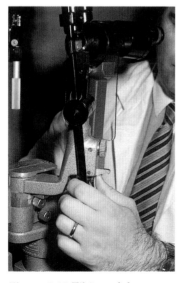

Figure 2.15 Tilting of the illumination column

Examination technique

1. Always tilt the illumination column (Figure 2.15) except when viewing the 12 o'clock position in the fundus (i.e. with the mirror at 6 o'clock).
2. When viewing horizontal meridians (i.e 3 and 9 o'clock positions in the fundus) keep the column central.
3. When viewing the vertical meridians (i.e 6 and 12 o'clock positions) the column can be left or right of centre (Figure 2.16).
4. When viewing oblique meridians (i.e 1.30 and 7.30 o'clock) keep the column right of centre, and vice versa when viewing the 10.30 and 4.30 o'clock positions.
5. When viewing different positions of the peripheral retina rotate the axis of the beam so that it is always at right angles to the mirror.
6. To visualize the entire fundus rotate the lens for 360° using first the equatorial mirror and then the peripheral mirror.

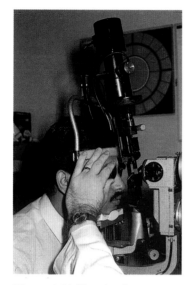

Figure 2.16 Illumination column tilted and positioned right of centre to view the oblique meridians at 1.30 o'clock and 7.30 o'clock

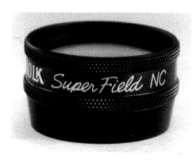

Figure 2.17 A wide field lens used for biomicroscopic indirect ophthalmoscopy

7. To obtain a more peripheral view of the retina tilt the lens to the opposite side and ask the patient to move the eyes to the same side. For example, to obtain a more peripheral view of 12 o'clock (with mirror at 6 o'clock) tilt the lens down and ask the patient to look up).
8. Examine the vitreous cavity with the central lens using both a horizontal and a vertical slit beam, and then examine the posterior pole.

Biomicroscopic indirect ophthalmoscopy

Slitlamp indirect ophthalmoscopy utilizes high power lenses (Figure 2.17) designed to obtain a wide field of view of the fundus. The lenses are used in a similar manner to an ordinary indirect ophthalmoscope lens and the image is also vertically inverted and laterally reversed. The technique is as follows:

1. Adjust the slitbeam to about 1/4 its full round diameter.
2. Set the illumination angle coaxial with the slitlamp viewing system.
3. Set the magnification and light intensity at their lowest settings.
4. Focus on the cornea and centre the light beam to pass directly through the patient's pupil.
5. Hold the lens directly in front of the cornea just clearing the lashes so that the light beam passes through its centre.
6. Examine the fundus by moving the joystick and vertical adjustment of the slitlamp but hold the lens still.
7. Reduce reflections by tilting or angling the light beam.
8. Increase the width of the beam to obtain a larger field of view.
9. Increase the magnification for greater detail as necessary.
10. To view the peripheral retina ask the patient to look into appropriate positions of gaze as with standard indirect ophthalmoscopy.

Interpretation of signs

1. The normal vitreous in a young individual appears homogeneous with the same density throughout. Swift ocular movements produce undulating folds in the gel and a few small opacities may be seen.
2. The central vitreous cavity contains optically empty spaces (lacunae). The condensed lining of a large cavity may be mistaken for a detached posterior hyaloid surface (pseudo-PVD).
3. In eyes with PVD the detached posterior hyaloid surface (Figure 2.18) can usually be traced to its insertion into the vitreous base above.

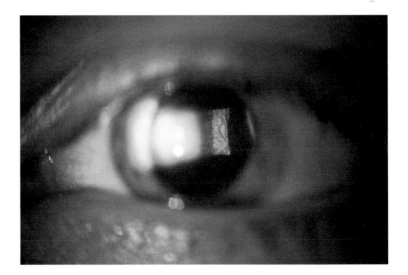

Figure 2.18 Posterior hyaloid face in an eye with posterior vitreous detachment

4. A Weiss' ring is an annular opacity representing a ring of glial tissue detached from the margin of the optic disc; it is virtually pathognomonic of PVD.
5. Pigment cells ('tobacco dust') in the retrolental space (Figure 2.19) in a patient complaining of sudden onset of flashing lights and floaters are strongly suggestive of a retinal tear. A careful examination of the peripheral retina (particularly superiorly) is mandatory. The cells consist of macrophages containing shed RPE cells.

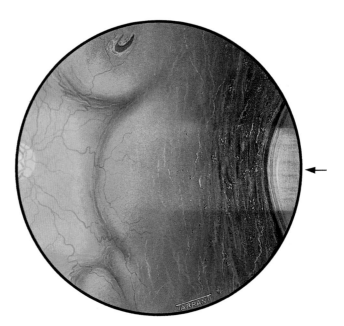

Figure 2.19 Tobacco dust in the anterior vitreous in an eye with a retinal detachment caused by a superior U-tear

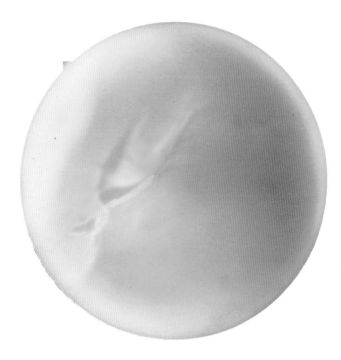

Figure 2.20 Two U-tears

6.   Numerous small opacities within the anteriorly displaced gel or in the retrohyaloid space are strongly suggestive of blood.
7.   Because of the wide field of view it may also be possible to visualize equatorial retinal tears (Figure 2.20).

How to find the primary retinal break

The primary break is defined as the one responsible for the RD. A secondary break is not responsible for the RD because it is either present before the development of RD or forms after RD has occurred. Finding the primary break is of paramount importance and aided by the following considerations.

Quadrantic distribution of breaks

The quadrantic distribution of breaks in eyes with RD is as follows: about 60% in the upper temporal quadrant; 15% in the upper nasal quadrant; 15% in the lower temporal quadrant; and 10% in the lower nasal quadrant. The upper temporal quadrant is therefore by far the most common site for retinal break formation and should be examined in great detail if a retinal break cannot be detected initially. It should also be remembered that

23

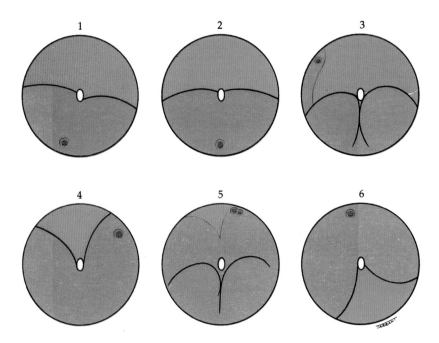

Figure 2.21 Shape of retinal detachment in relation to the primary break

about 50% of eyes with RD have more than one break, and in most eyes these are located within 90° of each other.

Configuration of SRF

SRF usually spreads in a gravitational fashion, and its shape is governed by anatomical limits (ora serrata and optic nerve) and the location of the primary retinal break. If the primary break is located superiorly, the SRF first spreads inferiorly on the same side as the break and then spreads superiorly on the opposite side of the fundus. The likely location of the primary retinal break can therefore be predicted by studying the shape of the RD (Figure 2.21).

1. A shallow inferior RD in which the SRF is slightly higher on the temporal side points to a primary break on that side.
2. A primary break located at 6 o'clock will cause an inferior RD with equal fluid levels.
3. In a bullous inferior RD the primary break usually lies above the horizontal meridian.
4. If the primary break is located in the upper nasal quadrant the SRF will revolve around the optic disc and then rise on the temporal side until it is level with the primary break.
5. A subtotal RD with a superior wedge of attached retina points to a primary break located in the periphery nearest its highest border.

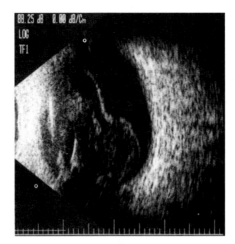

Figure 2.22 B-scan axial view showing an intragel haemorrhage and posterior vitreous detachment (courtesy of Mr K. Nischal)

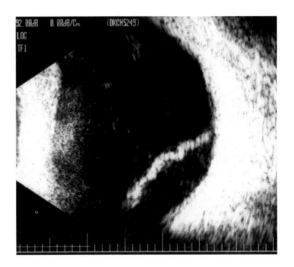

Figure 2.23 B-scan sagittal view showing an inferior retinal detachment (courtesy of Mr K. Nischal)

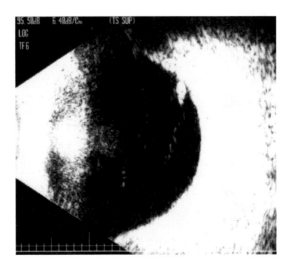

Figure 2.24 B-scan sagittal view showing a superior retinal tear associated with posterior vitreous detachment but a flat retina (courtesy of Mr K. Nischal)

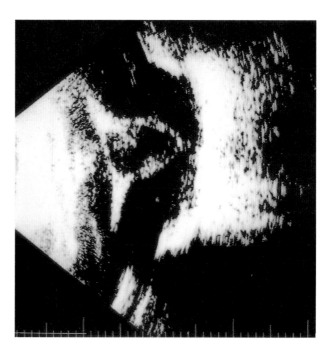

Figure 2.25 B-scan sagittal view showing the triangular sign of a total retinal detachment associated with advanced proliferative vitreoretinopathy (courtesy of Mr K. Nischal)

6. When the SRF crosses the vertical midline above, the primary break is near to 12 o'clock, the lower edge of the RD corresponding to the side of the break.

The above points are important because they prevent you from treating a secondary break and overlooking the primary break. It is therefore essential that you ensure that the shape of the RD corresponds to the location of the primary retinal break.

History

Although the quadrantic location of light flashes is of no value in predicting the location of the primary break, the quadrant in which the visual field defect first appears may be of considerable value. For example, if the field defect started in the upper nasal quadrant the primary break is probably located in the lower temporal quadrant.

Ultrasonography

B-scan ultrasonography is extremely useful in patients with opaque media suspected of having either a retinal tear or RD. This applies particularly in those with a recent dense vitreous haemorrhage which obscures visualization of the fundus. In these cases ultrasonography will help to differentiate a PVD (Figure 2.22) from a RD (Figure 2.23). It may also be possible to detect the presence of a retinal tear in flat retina (Figure 2.24). It is helpful if the surgeon is present at the ultrasound examination or performs it himself rather than relying on a photograph supplied with the report. Dynamic ultrasonography, in which examination of intraocular structures is performed during lateral eye movements, is helpful in assessing the mobility of the vitreous and retina in eyes with proliferative vitreoretinopathy (Figure 2.25).

3 Pathogenesis of retinal detachment

Rhegmatogenous retinal detachment
   Dynamic vitreoretinal traction
   Predisposing peripheral retinal degenerations
   Significance of myopia
   Significance of trauma

Tractional retinal detachment
   Diabetic tractional RD
   Traumatic tractional RD

Exudative retinal detachment

Rhegmatogenous retinal detachment

Rhegmatogenous RD affects about 1 in 10 000 of the population each year and both eyes are eventually involed in about 10% of cases. The retinal breaks responsible for RD are caused by an interplay between dynamic vitreoretinal traction and an

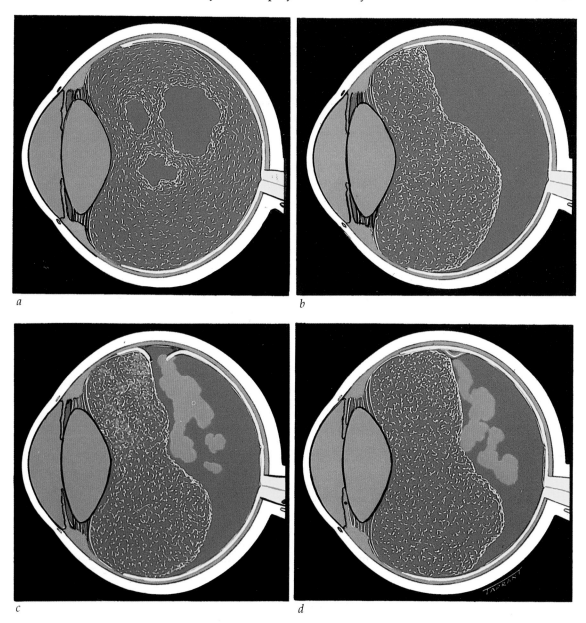

a   *b*

c   *d*

Figure 3.1 Acute posterior vitreous detachment. (*a*), synchisis; (*b*), uncomplicated posterior vitreous detachment; (*c*), retinal tear formation and vitreous haemorrhage; (*d*), avulsion of a retinal blood vessel and vitreous haemorrhage.

underlying weakness in the peripheral retina referred to as a **predisposing degeneration**.

Dynamic vitreoretinal traction

Pathogenesis

Synchysis is a liquefaction of the vitreous gel caused by alterations of its micromolecular structure (Figure 3.1*a*). Some eyes with synchysis develop a hole in the thinned posterior vitreous cortex which overlies the fovea. The synchytic fluid from within the centre of the vitreous cavity passes through this defect into the newly formed retrohyaloid space. This process forcibly detaches the posterior vitreous surface from the ILM of the sensory retina as far as the posterior border of the vitreous base. The remaining solid vitreous gel collapses inferiorly and the retrohyaloid space is occupied entirely by synchytic fluid. This process is called acute rhegmatogenous PVD with collapse and will be referred to as acute PVD henceforth.

Complications of acute PVD

Following PVD, the sensory retina is no longer protected by the stable vitreous cortex and can be directly affected by dynamic vitreoretinal tractional forces. The vision-threatening complications of acute PVD are dependent on the strength and extent of pre-existing vitreoretinal adhesions.

1. **No complications** occur in most eyes because vitreoretinal attachments are weak so that the vitreous cortex detaches completely without sequelae (Figure 3.1*b*).
2. **Retinal tears** develop in 10–15% of eyes as a result of transmission of traction at sites of abnormally strong vitreoretinal adhesions (Figure 3.1*c*). As previously mentioned these include:
   (a) 'White-without-pressure' (Figure 3.2*g*).
   (b) Retinal pigment clumps (Figure 3.2*h*).
   (c) Strong paravascular attachments (Figure 3.2*j*).
   (d) Posterior border of lattice degeneration (see Figure 3.6*c*).
   (e) Cystic retinal tufts.
   Although tears usually develop at the time of PVD, very occasionally they may be delayed by several weeks or even months. Tears associated with acute PVD are usually symptomatic, U-shaped, located in the upper fundus and frequently associated with vitreous haemorrhage resulting from rupture of a peripheral retinal blood vessel. After the tear has formed, the synchitic retrohyaloid fluid has direct access to the subretinal space. Unless the tear is treated prophylactically by photocoagulation or cryotherapy the risk of RD is high.

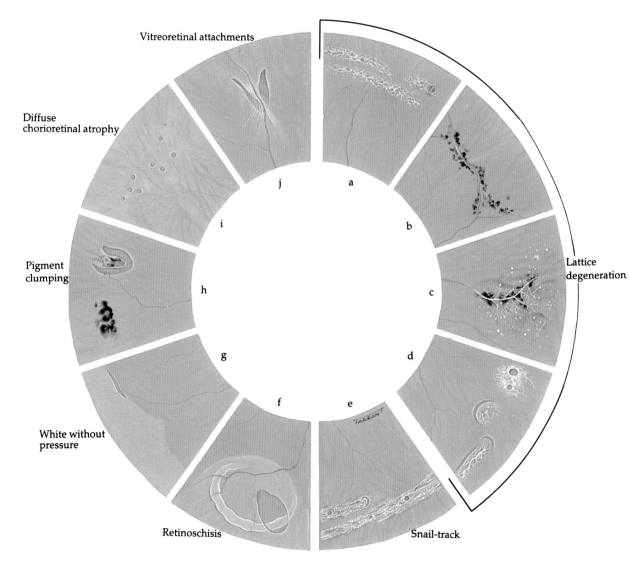

Figure 3.2 Predisposing peripheral retinal lesions

3. **Avulsion of a peripheral retinal blood vessel** resulting in vitreous haemorrhage in the absence of retinal tear formation is a rare complication (Figure 3.1*d*).

Predisposing peripheral retinal degenerations

About 60% of all breaks develop in areas of the peripheral retina that show specific changes. These lesions may be associated with a spontaneous breakdown of pathologically thin retinal tissue to cause a retinal hole, or they may predispose to retinal tear

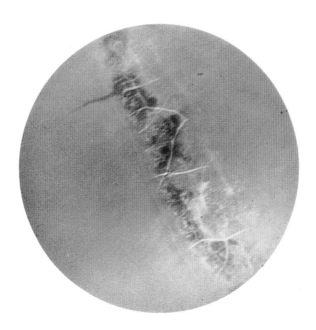

Figure 3.3 Typical lattice degeneration

formation in eyes with acute PVD. Retinal holes are round or oval in shape. They are usually smaller than tears and carry a lesser risk of RD.

Lattice degeneration

Lattice degeneration is present in about 8% of the general population. It probably develops early in life, with a peak incidence during the second and third decades. It is therefore not an age-related condition. Although lattice may be familial it shows no sexual predilection. It is found more commonly in moderate myopes and is the most important degeneration directly related to RD. It is present in about 40% of eyes with RD and is an important cause of RD in young myopes. Lattice-like lesions are frequently found in patients with Marfan's syndrome, Stickler's syndrome and Ehlers-Danlos syndrome, all of which are associated with an increased risk of RD.

Clinical features

1. **Typical lattice** consists of sharply demarcated, spindle-shaped areas of retinal thinning, most frequently located between the equator and the posterior border of the vitreous base. The condition is usually bilateral and more frequently located in the temporal than nasal half of the fundus, and superiorly rather than inferiorly. The islands of lattice may form two (Figure 3.2a), three or even four circumferentially oriented rows. A characteristic feature is an arborizing network of tiny white lines within the islands

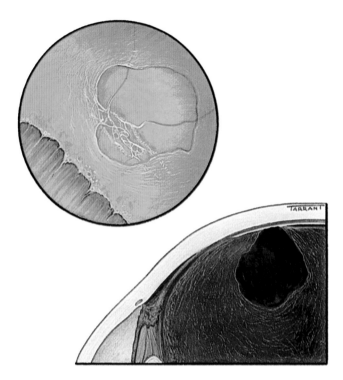

Figure 3.4 Vitreous changes associated with lattice degeneration

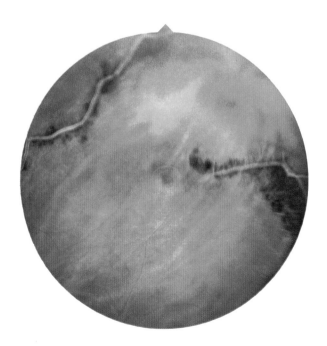

Figure 3.5 Atypical radial lattice degeneration in Stickler's syndrome

(Figure 3.3). The vitreous overlying an area of lattice is synchytic but the vitreous attachments around the margin of the lesion are exaggerated (Figure 3.4). Other features associated with lattice include:

    (a) Hyperplasia of the RPE (Figures 3.2*b*, 3.3).
    (b) 'Snowflakes' (Figure 3.2*c*).
    (c) 'White-with-pressure'.

2. **Atypical lattice** is characterized by radially orientated lesions continuous with peripheral blood vessels which may extend posterior to the equator (Figures 3.2*c*, 3.5, and 3.6*a*). This type typically occurs in patients with Stickler's syndrome.

Complications

1. **No complications** are encountered in most patients, even in the presence of small holes which are frequently found within islands of lattice (Figure 3.6*d*).
2. **RD associated with atrophic holes** may occasionally occur, particularly in young myopes. In these patients the RD may not be preceded by symptoms of acute PVD (photopsiae and floaters) and the SRF usually spreads slowly.
3. **RD associated with tractional tears** may occur in eyes with acute PVD. The tears typically develop along the posterior edge of an island of lattice as a result of dynamic traction at the site of an exaggerated vitreoretinal attachment. Occasionally a small island of lattice is present on the flap

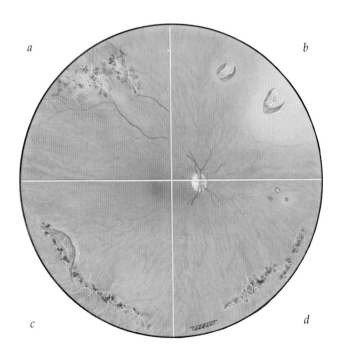

Figure 3.6 Lattice degeneration. (*a*), radial lattice degeneration; (*b*), lattice degeneration on the flap of a U-tear; (*c*), tractional tear along the posterior margin of lattice degeneration; (*d*), small round holes in lattice degeneration

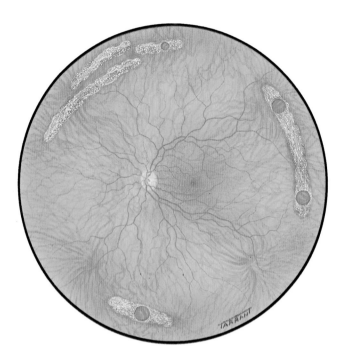

Figure 3.7 Snailtrack degeneration associated with large round holes

of a retinal tear (Figure 3.6*b*). RDs due to lattice tears typically occur in myopes over the age of 50 years; the SRF progresses more rapidly than in RDs caused by small round holes.

Snailtrack degeneration

Snailtrack degeneration is common in myopic eyes. It is characterized by sharply demarcated bands of tightly packed 'snowflakes' which give the peripheral retina a white frost-like appearance (Figure 3.7). Islands of snailtracks are usually longer than islands of lattice and may be associated with 'white-with-pressure'. Although snailtrack is associated with overlying vitreous liquefaction, marked vitreous traction at the posterior border of the lesions is seldom present so that tractional U-tears rarely occur. The characteristic lesion is a large round hole which carries a high risk of RD.

Degenerative retinoschisis

Retinoschisis is a splitting of the sensory retina into two layers – an outer (choroidal layer) and an inner (vitreous layer). The three main types are: (a) **congenital**, (b) **tractional** and (c) **degenerative**. Only the last type will be discussed.

Clinical features

Degenerative retinoschisis can be either **typical**, in which the split occurs at the outer plexiform layer, or the less common

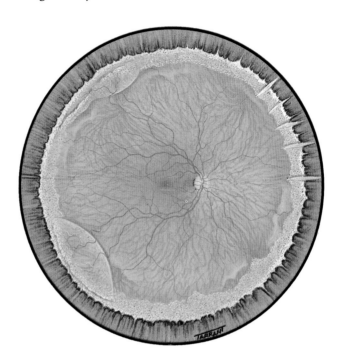

Figure 3.8 Degenerative retinoschisis involving the inferotemporal and superotemporal peripheral retina

reticular, in which the split is at the level of the nerve fibre layer. The condition is present in about 5% of the population over the age of 20 years and is particularly prevalent in hypermetropes (70% of patients are hypermetropic). Degenerative retinoschisis is almost always asymptomatic and in its early stages usually involves the extreme inferotemporal periphery of both fundi, appearing as an exaggeration of microcystoid degeneration with a smooth elevation of the retina (Figure 3.8). The lesion may progress circumferentially until it has involved the entire fundus periphery. The typical form usually remains anterior to the equator although the reticular type may spread beyond the equator and rarely threatens the fovea. The surface of the inner layer may show 'snowflakes' as well as sheathing or 'silver-wiring' of blood vessels (Figure 3.9). The outer layer has a beaten-metal appearance and shows the phenomenon of 'white-with-pressure'. The schisis cavity may be bridged by rows of torn grey-white tissue.

Complications

1. **No complications** occur in most cases and the condition is innocuous.
2. **Breaks** may develop in the reticular type. Inner layer breaks are small and round, whilst the less common outer layer breaks are usually larger, with rolled edges and located behind the equator (Figure 3.10, *left*). Eyes with only inner layer breaks do not develop RD as there is no communication with the subretinal space.

37

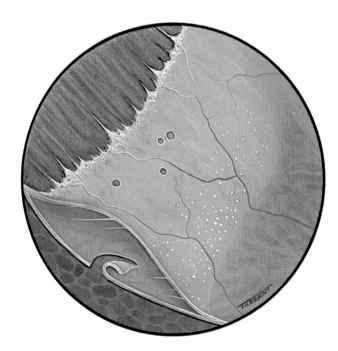

Figure 3.9 Degenerative retinoschisis with holes in both layers

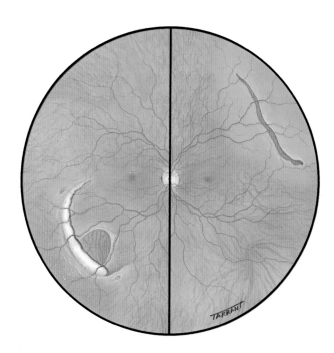

Figure 3.10 Degenerative retinoschisis. *Left:* large defects in both layers; *right:* large defect in the posterior layer associated with a localized retinal detachment

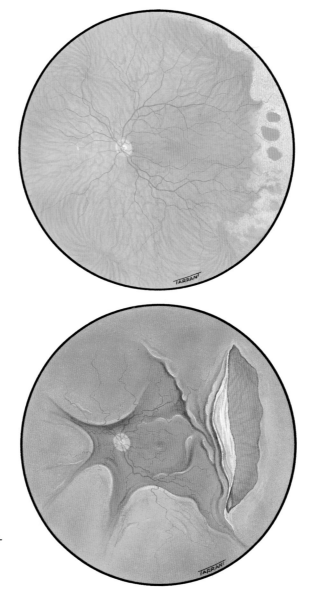

Figure 3.11 *Top:* 'white-without-pressure' involving temporal periphery with pseudoholes; *bottom:* giant retinal tear

3. **RD** is a very rare complication which may develop in eyes with breaks in both layers, especially in the presence of PVD. Eyes with only outer layer breaks do not as a rule develop RD because the fluid within the schisis cavity is viscous and does not pass readily into the subretinal space. Rarely, however, the schisis fluid loses its viscosity and passes through the break into the subretinal space, giving rise to a localized detachment of the outer retinal layer which is usually confined to the area of retinoschisis (Figure 3.10,

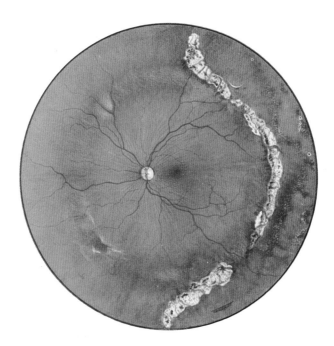

Figure 3.12 Appearance following prophylactic treatment of 'white-without-pressure' of a patient with a giant tear in the fellow eye

right). The detachment is almost always asymptomatic, infrequently progressive and rarely requires treatment.

4. **Vitreous haemorrhage** is an uncommon complication.

'White-without-pressure'

Clinical features

The phenomenon of 'white-*with*-pressure' is a translucent grey appearance of the retina, induced by indenting the sclera. Each area has a fixed configuration which does not change when the scleral indentor is moved to an adjacent area. In particularly marked cases the retina has the same appearance even without scleral indentation; this is termed 'white-*without*-pressure' (Figure 3.11, *top*). 'White-with-pressure' is frequently seen in normal eyes and may be observed along the posterior border of islands of lattice degeneration, snailtrack degeneration and outer layer of acquired retinoschisis. On cursory examination a normal area of retina surrounded by 'white-without-pressure' may be mistaken for a flat retinal hole.

Complications

Giant tears occasionally develop along the posterior border of 'white-without-pressure' (Figure 3.11, *bottom*). For this reason, if 'white-without-pressure' is found in the fellow eye of a patient with a spontaneous giant retinal tear, prophylactic therapy should be performed. However, it is advisable to treat all fellow eyes prophylactically irrespective of the presence of 'white-without-pressure' (Figure 3.12).

Diffuse chorioretinal atrophy

Diffuse chorioretinal atrophy is characterized by choroidal depigmentation and thinning of the overlying retina in the equatorial area of highly myopic eyes (see Figure 3.2*i*). Retinal holes developing in the atrophic retina may lead to RD. Because of lack of contrast between the depigmented choroid and sensory retina, small holes may be very difficult to visualize without the help of slitlamp examination as previously described.

Significance of myopia

Although myopes make up 10% of the general population, over 40% of all RDs occur in myopic eyes. The higher the refractive error the greater the risk of RD. The following interrelated factors predispose a myopic eye to RD:

1. **Lattice degeneration** is more common in moderate myopes and may give rise to either tractional tears or trophic holes.
2. **Snailtrack degeneration** is common in myopic eyes and may be associated with large trophic holes.
3. **Diffuse chorioretinal atrophy** may give rise to small round holes in highly myopic eyes.
4. **Macular holes** may give rise to RD in highly myopic eyes.
5. **Vitreous degeneration** and PVD are more common.
6. **Vitreous loss** during cataract surgery, particularly if inappropriately managed, is associated with about a 15% incidence of subsequent RD in myopic eyes greater than 6D; the risk is even higher if myopia is more than 10D.
7. **Posterior capsulotomy** is associated with an increased risk of RD in myopic eyes, particularly if performed within one year of cataract surgery.

Significance of trauma

Trauma is responsible for about 10% of all cases of RD and is the most common cause in children, particularly boys. A great variety of breaks may develop in traumatized eyes either at the time of impact or subsequently. Eyes with penetrating injuries of the posterior segment are at particular risk of RD, particularly if there is vitreous incarceration at the site of penetration.

Severe blunt ocular trauma causes a compression of the antero-posterior diameter of the globe and a simultaneous expansion at the equatorial plane. The relatively inelastic vitreous gel causes traction along the posterior aspect of the vitreous base with tearing of the retina to form a dialysis (Figure 3.13). In some cases the vitreous base becomes avulsed giving rise to a 'bucket-handle' appearance (Figure 3.14) which comprises a strip of

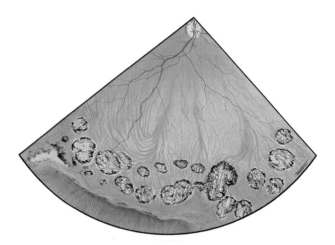

Figure 3.13 Appearance following prophylactic cryotherapy to a traumatic retinal dialysis unassociated with retinal detachment

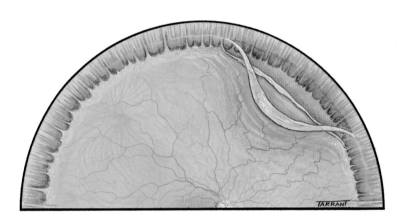

Figure 3.14 Traumatic retinal dialysis with the characteristic 'bucket handle' appearance of the avulsed vitreous base

ciliary epithelium, ora serrata and the immediate post-oral retina into which basal vitreous gel remains inserted. Traumatic dialyses may occur in any quadrant but are more frequent in the upper nasal. Although they occur at the time of injury, the RD usually does not develop until several months later. Progression is frequently slow, probably because the vitreous gel is healthy in a young individual. Other less common post-contusive breaks are macular and equatorial holes. The latter often occur at the site of scleral impact (direct retinal injury). In extreme cases there is complete disruption of the retina and choroid with subsequent overgrowth of fibrous tissue (retinitis sclopetaria).

Tractional retinal detachment

The main causes of tractional RD are: (a) **proliferative diabetic retinopathy**, (b) **retinopathy of prematurity**, (c) **proliferative**

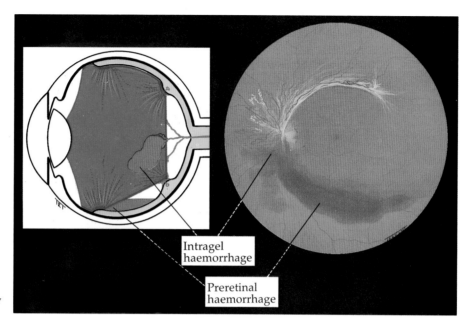

Figure 3.15
Incomplete
posterior vitreous
detachment in
severe proliferative
diabetic retinopathy

sickle cell retinopathy and (d) **penetrating posterior segment trauma.**

Diabetic tractional RD

Pathogenesis of PVD

Tractional RD is a devastating complication of proliferative diabetic retinopathy. It is caused by progressive contraction of fibrovascular membranes over large areas of vitreoretinal adhesion. In contrast to acute PVD in eyes with rhegmatogenous RD, PVD in diabetic eyes is gradual, non-rhegmatogenous and frequently incomplete. It is thought to be caused by leakage of plasma constituents into the vitreous gel from a fibrovascular network, which becomes adherent to the posterior vitreous surface. Owing to the strong adhesions of the cortical vitreous to areas of fibrovascular proliferation, PVD is usually incomplete (Figure 3.15). In the very rare event of a complete PVD, the new blood vessels are avulsed and RD does not develop.

Vitreoretinal traction

The following three main types of static vitreoretinal traction are recognized.

1. **Tangential** traction is caused by the contraction of epiretinal fibrovascular membranes with puckering of the retina and distortion of retinal blood vessels (Figure 3.16).

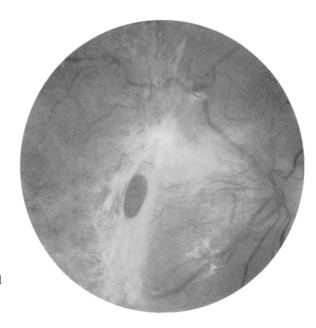

Figure 3.16 Distortion of retinal blood vessels resulting from tangential contraction of fibrovascular tissue in advanced proliferative diabetic retinopathy

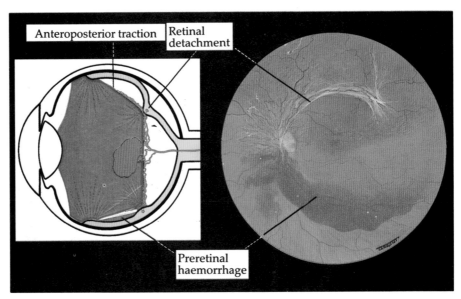

Figure 3.17 Anteroposterior vitreoretinal traction giving rise to a superior tractional retinal detachment in advanced proliferative diabetic retinopathy

2. **Anteroposterior** traction is caused by the contraction of fibrovascular membranes extending from the posterior retina, usually in association with the major arcades, to the vitreous base anteriorly (Figure 3.17).

3. **Bridging (trampoline)** traction is the result of contraction of fibrovascular membranes which stretch from one part of the posterior retina to another (Figure 3.18). This tends to pull the two involved points together and may be responsible for

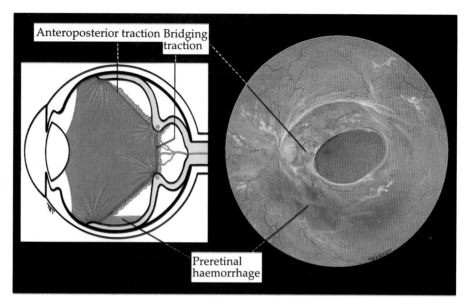

Anteroposterior traction Bridging traction

Preretinal haemorrhage

Figure 3.18
Bridging and anteroposterior vitreoretinal traction giving rise to an extensive tractional retinal detachment in advanced proliferative diabetic retinopathy

the formation of stress lines as well as displacement of the macula towards the disc or elsewhere depending on the direction of traction. Occasionally, vitreoretinal traction causes tractional retinoschisis rather than RD. In some eyes, incomplete avulsion of a portion of a fibrovascular membrane gives rise to a retinal tear (usually small and posterior to the equator). When this happens, the characteristic shape of a tractional RD assumes the configuration of a rhegmatogenous RD and is referred to as a combined traction-rhegmatogenous RD.

Traumatic tractional RD

Traumatic tractional RD is the result of vitreous incarceration in the wound and the presence of blood within the vitreous gel which acts as a stimulus to fibroblastic proliferation along the planes of incarcerated vitreous. The contraction of such anterior epiretinal membranes leads to a shortening and a rolling effect on the peripheral retina in the region of the vitreous base and eventually to an anterior tractional RD. A retinal break may develop several weeks later leading to a sudden extension of SRF and consequent visual loss. As a rule, in penetrating trauma the traction is therefore mainly anterior whereas in diabetes it is mainly posterior.

Exudative retinal detachment

Exudative (serous, secondary) RD is much less common than both rhegmatogenous and tractional. It is caused by subretinal disorders which damage the RPE and thereby allow the passage of fluid derived from the choroid into the subretinal space. A more correct description would therefore be 'transudative'. The main causes of exudative RDs are the following:

1. **Choroidal tumours** such as melanomas, haemangiomas and metastases. It is important always to consider that RD is caused by an intraocular tumour until proved otherwise.
2. **Inflammation** such as Harada's disease and posterior scleritis.
3. **Bullous central serous choroidopathy** is a rare cause.
4. **Iatrogenic** causes include retinal detachment surgery and panretinal photocoagulation. Postoperative exudative RD should not be mistaken for a recurrence of a rhegmatogenous RD (see Chapter 9).
5. **Subretinal neovascularization** which may leak and give rise to extensive subretinal accumulation of fluid at the posterior pole.
6. **Hypertensive choroidopathy** which may occur in toxaemia of pregnancy is now a very rare cause.
7. **Idiopathic** such as that associated with the uveal effusion syndrome.

Treatment of exudative RDs depends on the cause. Some resolve spontaneously (postoperative), whilst others are treated with systemic corticosteroids (Harada's disease and posterior scleritis). In some eyes with central serous choroidopathy the leak in the RPE can be sealed by argon laser photocoagulation.

Further reading

Ambler, J. S., Gass, J. D. M. and Gutman, F. A. (1991) Symptomatic retinoschisis-detachment involving the macula. *American Journal of Ophthalmology*, **112**, 8–14

Byer, N. E. (1979) Lattice degeneration of the retina. *Survey of Ophthalmology*, **23**, 213-248

Celorio, J. M. and Pruett, R. C. (1991) Prevalence of lattice degeneration and its relationship to axial length in severe myopia. *American Journal of Ophthalmology*, **111**, 20–23

Cousins, S., Boniuk, I., Okun, E. *et al.* (1986) Pseudophakic retinal detachments in the presence of various intraocular lens types. *Ophthalmology*, **93**, 1198–1208

Dumas, J. and Schepens, C. L. (1966) Chorioretinal lesions predisposing to retinal breaks. *American Journal of Ophthalmology*, **61**, 620–630

Ficker, L. A., Vickers, S., Capon, M. R. C. *et al.* (1987) Retinal detachment following Nd:YAG laser posterior capsulotomy. *Eye*, **1**, 86–89

Foos, R. Y. and Wheeler, N. C. (1982) Vitreoretinal juncture. Synchisis senilis and posterior vitreous detachment. *Ophthalmology*, **89**, 1502–1512

Foulds, W. S. (1975) Aetiology of retinal detachment. *Transactions of the Ophthalmological Society of the UK*, **95**, 118–128

Gregor, Z. and Ryan, S. J. (1982) Combined posterior contusion and penetrating injury in the pig eye. II. Histological features. *British Journal of Ophthalmology*, **66**, 799–804

Grey, R. H., Evans, A. R., Constable, I. J. *et al.* (1989) Retinal detachment and its relation to cataract surgery. *British Journal of Ophthalmology,* **73,** 775–780

Johnston, P. B. (1991) Traumatic retinal detachment. *British Journal of Ophthalmology,* **75,** 18–21

Kanski, J. J. (1975) Complications of acute posterior vitreous detachment. *American Journal of Ophthalmology,* **80,** 44–46

Seward, H. C. and Doran, R. M. L. (1984) Posterior capsulotomy and retinal detachment following extracapsular lens surgery. *British Journal of Ophthalmology,* **68,** 379–382

Smith, P. W., Stark, W. J., Maumenee, A. E. *et al.* (1987) Retinal detachment after extracapsular cataract extraction with posterior chamber intraocular lens. *Ophthalmology,* **94,** 495–504

4 Clinical features of retinal detachment

Rhegmatogenous retinal detachment

Symptoms

The classic premonitory symptoms reported in about 60% of patients with spontaneous rhegmatogenous RD are flashing lights and vitreous floaters caused by acute PVD with collapse. After a variable period of time the patient notices a relative peripheral visual field defect which may progress to involve central vision.

Photopsia

Photopsia is a subjective sensation perceived as a flash of light. In eyes with acute PVD it is probably caused by traction at sites of vitreoretinal adhesion. The cessation of photopsia is the result of either separation of the adhesion or complete tearing away of a piece of retina (operculum) around the site of adhesion. In eyes with PVD the photopsia may be induced by eye movements and is more noticeable in dim illumination. It tends to be projected into the patient's temporal peripheral visual field and, unlike floaters, it has no lateralizing value. Photopsia caused by vitreoretinal traction should be differentiated from migraine.

Floaters

A floater is a moving vitreous opacity which is perceived when it casts a shadow onto the retina. Vitreous opacities in eyes with acute PVD are of the following three types:

1. A solitary ring-shaped opacity representing the detached annular attachment to the margin of the optic disc (Weiss' ring).
2. Cobwebs are caused by condensation of collagen fibres within the collapsed vitreous cortex.
3. A sudden shower of minute red-coloured or dark spots usually indicates vitreous haemorrhage secondary to tearing of a peripheral retinal blood vessel. Although vitreous haemorrhage associated with acute PVD is usually sparse because the bleeding blood vessel has a small calibre due to its peripheral location, occasionally a severe bleed may impair visualization of the fundus.

Visual field defect

A visual field defect is caused by spread of SRF behind the equator. It is perceived by the patient as a 'black curtain' which is usually progressive. In some patients it may not be present on waking in the morning due to spontaneous absorption of SRF, only to reappear later in the day. A lower field defect is usually appreciated more quickly by the patient than an upper field defect. The quadrant of the visual field in which the field defect

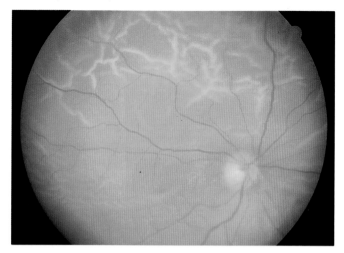

Figure 4.1 Fresh retinal detachment with the characteristic corrugated appearance caused by intraretinal oedema

first appears is useful in predicting the location of the primary retinal break (which will be in the opposite quadrant). Loss of central vision may be due either to involvement of the fovea by SRF or, less frequently, obstruction of the visual axis by a large upper bullous RD.

Signs

1. A Marcus Gunn pupil (relative afferent pupillary defect) is present in eyes with extensive RDs irrespective of the type.
2. The intraocular pressure is usually lower by about 5 mmHg as compared with the normal eye. If the intraocular pressure is extremely low, an associated choroidal detachment may be present. If a patient with known pre-existing primary open-angle glaucoma develops a sudden drop of intraocular pressure the possibility of RD should be excluded and conversely if an eye with an extensive RD has normal intraocular pressure, the presence of primary open-angle glaucoma, which coexists with RD in about 5% of patients, should be suspected.
3. A mild iritis is very common. Occasionally it may be severe enough to cause posterior synechiae. In these cases the underlying RD may be overlooked and the poor visual acuity incorrectly ascribed to some other cause.
4. The retrolental vitreous shows 'tobacco dust' as previously described (see Figure 2.19).
5. The retinal signs depend on the duration of RD and the presence or absence of proliferative vitreoretinopathy. Retinal breaks appear as discontinuities in the retinal surface. They are usually red because of the colour contrast between the sensory retina and underlying choroid. However, in eyes with hypopigmented choroid (as in high myopia), the colour contrast is decreased and small breaks may be overlooked unless careful slitlamp examination is performed.

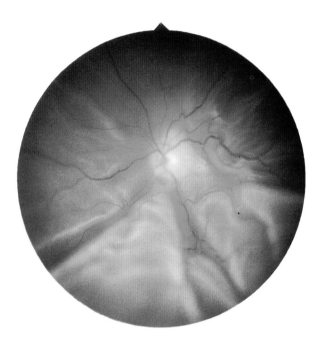

Figure 4.2 Total retinal detachment

Fresh retinal detachment

The detached retina has a convex configuration and a slightly opaque and corrugated appearance as a result of intraretinal oedema (Figures 4.1, 4.2). There is loss of the underlying choroidal pattern and retinal blood vessels appear darker than in flat retina, so the colour contrast between venules and arterioles is less apparent (Figure 4.3). The SRF extends up to the ora serrata except in the rare cases caused by a macular hole in which the SRF is initially confined to the posterior pole. The detached retina undulates freely with eye movements. Because of the thinness of the retina at the fovea, a pseudohole is frequently seen if the posterior pole is detached. This should not be mistaken for a true macular hole which may give rise to RD in highly myopic eyes or following blunt ocular trauma (Figure 4.4).

Long-standing retinal detachment

The following are the main features of a long-standing rhegmatogenous RD which do not occur in any other type irrespective of duration (Figure 4.5):

1. **Retinal thinning** secondary to atrophy is a characteristic finding which must not be mistaken for retinoschisis.
2. **Secondary intraretinal cysts** may develop if the RD has been present for about one year. They tend to disappear after retinal reattachment.

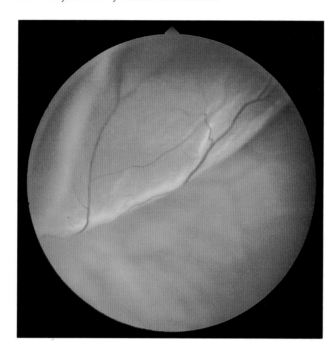

Figure 4.3 Fresh superior bullous retinal detachment

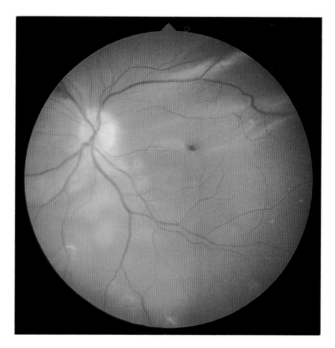

Figure 4.4 Shallow retinal detachment caused by a traumatic macular hole

3. **Subretinal demarcation lines** (high water marks) caused by proliferation of RPE cells at the junction of flat and detached retina are common and take about 3 months to develop. They are initially pigmented (Figure 4.6, *right*) and then tend to lose their pigment. Demarcation lines are convex with respect to

53

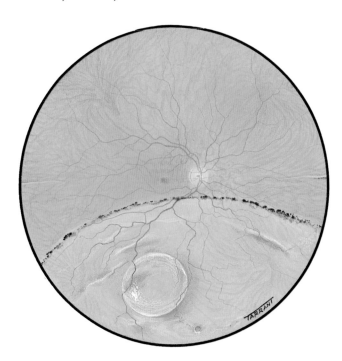

Figure 4.5 Long-standing inferior retinal detachment associated with a secondary intraretinal cyst and a pigmented demarcation line

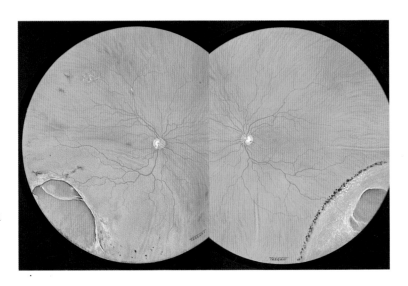

Figure 4.6 Bilateral long-standing inferotemporal retinal detachments resulting from dialyses. *Left:* unassociated with a demarcation line; *right:* associated with a pigmented demarcation line

the ora serrata and, although they represent sites of increased adhesion, they do not invariably limit spread of SRF.

4. **Peripheral neovascularization** may occasionally be present.

Proliferative vitreoretinopathy

Proliferative vitreoretinopathy (PVR) is caused by the proliferation of membranes on the inner retinal surface (epiretinal

54

membranes), on the posterior surface of the detached hyaloid and occasionally also on the outer retinal surface (subretinal membranes). These membranes are thought to be caused by the proliferation and metaplasia of cells derived from the RPE and retinal glia. Mild PVR is found in about 5% of eyes with RD and can be managed successfully with standard scleral buckling procedures. In some eyes contraction of the fibrous component of epiretinal and, sometimes, subretinal membranes causes tangential traction with varying degrees of distortion of affected retina. Severe postoperative contraction of tangential membranes and transvitreal membranes is the most common cause of failure in RD surgery requiring vitreoretinal surgery.

The main clinical features of PVR are retinal folds and rigidity so that retinal mobility induced by eye movements or scleral indentation is decreased according to severity. The following is the classification of PVR, but it should be emphasized that progression from one stage to the next is not inevitable.

Grade A (minimal) PVR is characterized by diffuse vitreous haze and 'tobacco dust'. There may also be pigmented cells on the inferior surface of the retina. Although these findings occur in many eyes with RD, they are particularly severe in eyes with early PVR.

Grade B (moderate) PVR is characterized by wrinkling of the inner retinal surface, tortuosity of blood vessels, retinal stiffness, decreased mobility of vitreous gel and rolled and irregular edges of retinal breaks (Figure 4.7). The epiretinal membranes

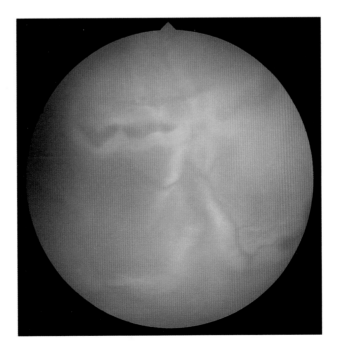

Figure 4.7 Rolled edges of retinal tears in Grade B proliferative vitreoretinopathy

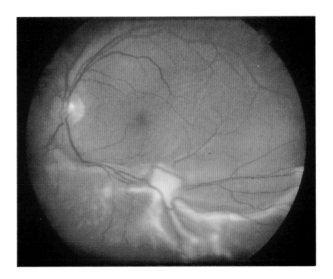

Figure 4.8 Posterior
proliferative vitreoretinopathy
Grade C-Type 1 characterized
by focal starfold contraction

responsible for these findings cannot be identified by indirect
ophthalmoscopy.

Grade C (marked) PVR is characterized by full-thickness rigid
retinal folds with heavy vitreous condensation and strands. It
can be either anterior (A) or posterior (P), the rough dividing
line being the equator of the globe. The severity of proliferation
in each area is expressed by the number of clock hours of retina

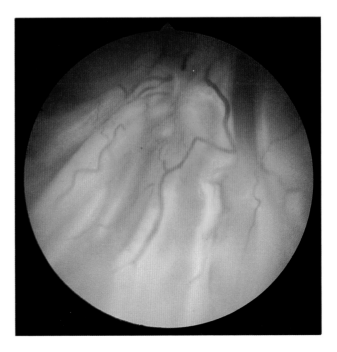

Figure 4.9 Posterior
proliferative vitreoretinopathy
Grade C-Type 2 characterized
by diffuse contraction with
confluent starfolds

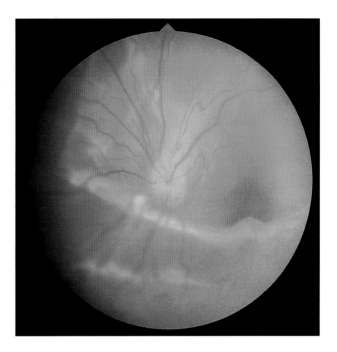

Figure 4.10 Posterior proliferative vitreoretinopathy Grade C-Type 3 characterized by subretinal proliferation

involved (1-12), although proliferations need not be contiguous. The type of contraction is further described as: (a) type 1 (focal), (b) type 2 (diffuse), (c) type 3 (subretinal), (d) type 4 (circumferential) and (e) type 5 (anterior displacement).

Grade C-P is therefore subdivided into the following three types:

1. Focal contraction with star folds posterior to the vitreous base (type 1) (Figure 4.8 and see Figure 8.36).
2. Diffuse contraction with confluent starfolds (type 2) (Figure 4.9).
3. Subretinal proliferation (type 3) (Figures 4.10, 4.11).

Grade C-A is subdivided as follows:

1. Subretinal proliferation (type 3).
2. Circumferentail contraction along posterior border of vitreous base (type 4).
3. Vitreous base is pulled anteriorly by proliferative tissue (type 5).

Subsequent course of untreated RD

1. **Progression** occurs in most cases. The RD becomes total and eventually gives rise to secondary cataract, chronic uveitis, hypotony and eventually phthisis bulbi.
2. **Non-progression** occurs in a minority of cases. The RD remain stationary for many years or indefinitely due to the formation of demarcation lines.

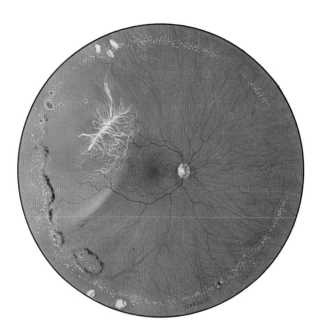

Figure 4.11 Subretinal
membrane proliferation

3. **Regression** is very rare but a small RD may reattach sponta-
    neously, particularly if the patient is subjected to prolonged
    bed rest.

Tractional retinal detachment

Symptoms

Photopsia and floaters are usually absent because vitreoretinal
traction develops insidiously and is not associated with acute
PVD. The visual field defect usually progresses slowly and may
become stationary for months and even years.

Signs

The detached retina has a concave configuration and breaks are
absent (Figure 4.12). The SRF is less than in a rhegmatogenous
RD and seldom extends to the ora serrata. The highest elevation
of the retina occurs at sites of vitreoretinal traction. Retinal
mobility is severely reduced and shifting fluid is absent. PVD is
present but incomplete. If a tractional RD develops a break it
assumes the characteristics of a rhegmatogenous RD and
progresses more quickly (combined tractional-rhegmatogenous
RD) (Figure 4.13).

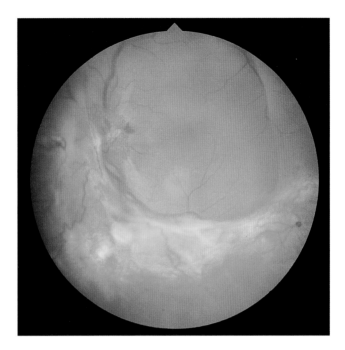

Figure 4.12 Tractional retinal detachment in advanced proliferative diabetic retinopathy

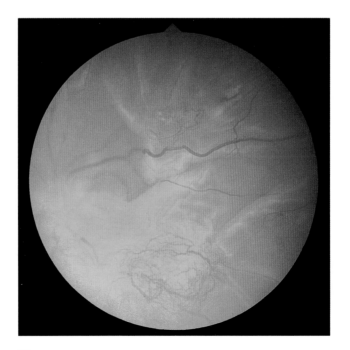

Figure 4.13 Combined diabetic tractional-rhegmatogenous retinal detachment showing a convex bullous configuration associated with retinal neovascularization

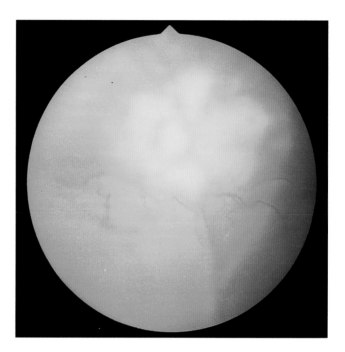

Figure 4.14 Exudative inferior
retinal detachment

Exudative retinal detachment

Symptoms

Photopsia is absent because there is no vitreoretinal traction
although floaters may be present if there is associated vitritis.
The visual field defect may develop suddenly and progress
rapidly. In some cases of Harada's disease both eyes are
involved simultaneously.

Signs

Retinal breaks are absent and the detached retina has a convex
configuration, just like a rhegmatogenous RD, but its surface is
smooth and not corrugated (Figure 4.14). Occasionally the SRF
is so deep that the RD can be seen with the slitlamp without the
aid of a contact lens, and it may even touch the back of the lens.
The detached retina is very mobile and shows the phenomenon
of 'shifting fluid' in which SRF responds to the force of gravity
and detaches the area of retina under which it accumulates. For
example, in the upright position the SRF collects under the
inferior retina but on assuming the supine position the inferior
retina flattens and the SRF shifts posteriorly and detaches the
macula and superior retina. Scattered areas of subretinal clump-
ing gives rise to the characteristic 'leopard spot' appearance may
be seen (Figure 4.15) and in eyes with posterior scleritis the SRF

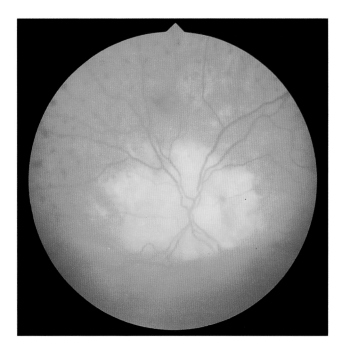

Figure 4.15 Same eye as in Figure 4.14 showing 'leopard spots' in superior fundus

may be turbid. The cause of the RD, such as a choroidal tumour, may be apparent when the fundus is examined, or the patient may have an associated systemic disease responsible for the RD (rheumatoid arthritis, Harada's disease, toxaemia, etc.).

Differential diagnosis of retinal detachment

Degenerative retinoschisis

Symptoms

Photopsia and floaters are absent because there is no vitreoretinal traction. A visual field defect is seldom observed because spread posterior to the equator is rare. If present it is absolute and not relative as in a RD. Occasionally symptoms occur as a result of either vitreous haemorrhage or development of progressive RD.

Signs

Breaks may be present in one or both layers in eyes with reticular retinoschisis. The elevation is convex, smooth, thin and relatively immobile unlike the opaque and corrugated appearance

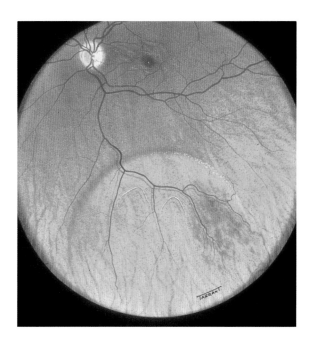

Figure 4.16 Degenerative retinoschisis with two outer layer breaks and 'snowflakes' on the inner layer

of a rhegmatogenous RD (Figure 4.16). The thin inner leaf of the schisis cavity may be mistaken, on cursory examination, for an atrophic long-standing rhegmatogenous RD but demarcation lines and secondary cysts in the inner leaf are absent.

Choroidal detachment

Symptoms

Photopsia and floaters are absent because there is no vitreoretinal traction and a visual field defect is seldom noticed.

Signs

The intraocular pressure may be very low as a result of concomitant detachment of the ciliary body. The anterior chamber is usually of normal depth but may be shallow in eyes with extensive choroidal detachments. The brown elevations are convex, smooth, bullous and relatively immobile. Temporal and nasal bullae tend to be most prominent (Figure 4.17). Because the detachments are limited anteriorly only by the scleral spur, the peripheral retina and ora serrata can be seen with ease without scleral indentation. The elevations do not extend to the posterior pole because they are limited by the firm adhesion between the

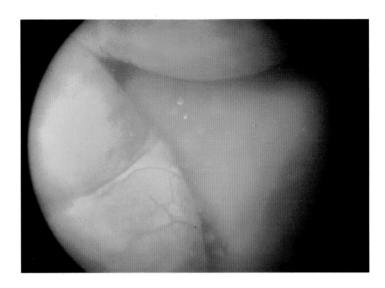

Figure 4.17 Choroidal detachments

suprachoroidal lamellae where the vortex veins enter their scleral canals.

Uveal effusion syndrome

The uveal effusion syndrome is characterized by choroidal detachments associated with an exudative RD (Figure 4.18).

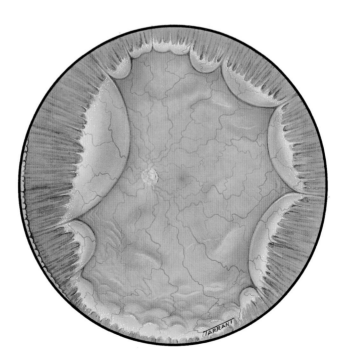

Figure 4.18 Uveal effusion syndrome characterized by choroidal detachments associated with an exudative retinal detachment

Following resolution the RPE frequently shows a characteristic residual mottling. It is a rare, idiopathic condition which may be mistaken for either a RD complicated by choroidal detachment or a ring malignant melanoma of the anterior choroid.

Further reading

Machemer, R., Aaberg, T. M., MacKenzie Freeman, H. *et al.* (1991) An updated classification of retinal detachment with proliferative vitreo-retinopathy. *American Journal of Ophthalmology*, **112**, 159–165

5 Prophylaxis of rhegmatogenous retinal detachment

Indications for prophylaxis

Retinal breaks

Although, given the right circumstances, most retinal breaks can cause RD, some are more dangerous than others. Important criteria to be considered in the selection of patients for prophylactic treatment can be divided into: (a) **characteristics of the break** and (b) **other considerations**.

Characteristics of the break

1. **Type**: a tear is more dangerous than a hole because it is associated with dynamic vitreoretinal traction.
2. **Size**: the larger the break the more dangerous.
3. **Symptomatic** tears associated with acute PVD are more dangerous than those detected on routine examination.
4. **Location** is important for the following reasons:
   (a) Superior are more dangerous than inferior breaks because, as a result of gravity, SRF is likely to spread more quickly. Supero-temporal tears are particularly dangerous because the macula is threatened early in the event of RD.
   (b) Equatorial are more dangerous than oral because the latter are usually located within the vitreous base.
5. **'Subclinical RD'** refers to a break surrounded by a small amount of SRF. As the SRF is usually located anterior to the equator it does not give rise to a peripheral visual field defect. 'Subclinical RDs' are dangerous because they may become 'clinical' within a short period of time.
6. **Pigmentation** around a retinal break indicates that it has been present for a long time and the danger of progression to clinical RD is small.

Other considerations

1. **Aphakia**: a retinal break in an aphakic eye is more dangerous than an identical lesion in a phakic eye. Even a relatively innocuous small peripheral round hole may give rise to RD following cataract extraction, particularly if associated with vitreous loss.
2. **Myopia**: as myopic patients are more prone to RD, a retinal break in a myopic eye should be taken more seriously than an identical lesion in a non-myopic eye.
3. **Only eye**: retinal breaks should be taken very seriously, particularly if the fellow eye has lost vision from RD.
4. **Family history**: any break or predisposing degeneration should be taken seriously if the patient gives a family history of RD.
5. **Systemic diseases** that are associated with an increased risk of RD are Marfan's syndrome, Stickler's syndrome and Ehlers–Danlos syndrome. As RD in these patients has a

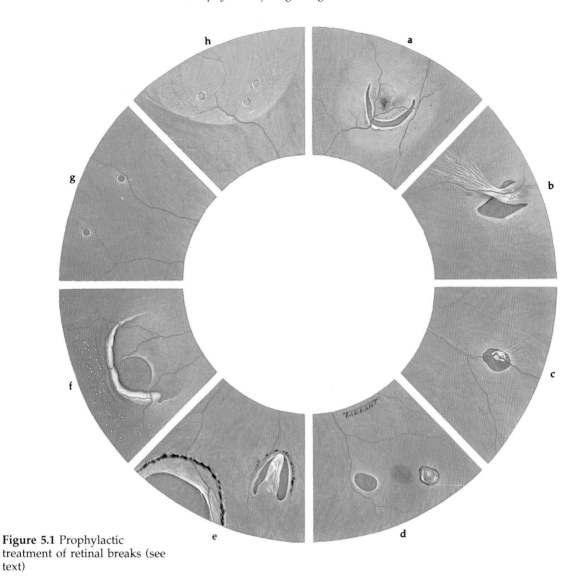

Figure 5.1 Prophylactic treatment of retinal breaks (see text)

relatively poor prognosis, any break or predisposing degeneration should be treated prophylactically.

Clinical examples

The following clinical examples illustrate the various risk factors just discussed (Figure 5.1):

1. A large equatorial U-tear associated with 'subclinical RD' and located in the upper temporal quadrant (Figure 5.1*a*) should be treated prophylactically without delay because the risk of progression to a clinical RD is very high. As the tear is located

in the upper temporal quadrant, early macular involvement by SRF is likely. Treatment should involve cryotherapy combined with an explant because this has the greatest chance of success. Argon laser photocoagulation alone is less appropriate because the break is surrounded by SRF.

2. A large U-tear in the upper temporal quadrant in an eye with symptomatic acute PVD (Figure 5.1b) should also be treated without delay because the risk of progression to clinical RD is high. Although the tear is not associated with a 'subclinical RD' it is still dangerous because it is large, in the upper temporal quadrant and symptomatic. Fresh tears such as this in patients with symptoms of acute PVD often progress to clinical RD within a few days or weeks unless treated prophylactically. In addition SRF accumulates more quickly in eyes with PVD because the volume of syneretic fluid is greater than in eyes with atrophic holes or dialyses without PVD. Treatment is by cryotherapy or laser photocoagulation. Because vitreoretinal traction is still present on the flap of the tear a local explant should also be considered.

3. An operculated U-tear bridged by a patent blood vessel (Figure 5.1c) should be treated because persistent dynamic vitreoretinal traction on the bridging blood vessel may cause recurrent vitreous haemorrhage. Although eyes with breaks associated with avulsed or bridging blood vessels may be successfully treated by argon laser photocoagulation alone, the possibility of an explant to reduce traction on the operculum and blood vessel should be considered.

4. A U-tear with a free-floating operculum in the lower temporal quadrant detected by chance (Figure 5.1d) is much safer because there is no vitreoretinal traction. Prophylaxis is therefore not required in the absence of other risk factors.

5. An inferior U-tear and a dialysis surrounded by pigment detected by chance (Figure 5.1e) are both low risk lesions which have been present for a long time. However, the presence of pigmentation around a large U-tear is not always a guarantee against progression, particularly when associated with other risk factors such as aphakia, myopia or RD in the fellow eye. If necessary, treatment can be with either cryotherapy or photocoagulation.

6. Degenerative retinoschisis with breaks in both layers (Figure 5.1f) does not require treatment. Although this lesion represents a full-thickness defect in the sensory retina, the fluid within the schisis cavity is usually viscid and rarely passes into the subretinal space.

7. Two small asymptomatic holes near the ora serrata (Figure 5.1g) do not require treatment because the risk of RD is extremely small as they are probably located within the vitreous base. About 5% of the general population have such lesions.

8. Small inner layer holes in retinoschisis (Figure 5.1h) also carry an extremely low risk of RD as there is no communication between the vitreous cavity and the subretinal space. Treatment is therefore inappropriate.

Predisposing peripheral retinal degenerations

In the absence of associated retinal breaks neither lattice nor snailtrack degenerations require prophylactic treatment unless they are associated with one or more of the following risk factors:

1. **RD in the fellow eye** is the most frequent indication.
2. **Aphakia or pseudophakia**, particularly if laser posterior capsulotomy is necessary.
3. **High myopia**, particularly if associated with extensive lattice degeneration.
4. **Strong family history of RD**.
5. **Systemic disease** known to predispose to RD such as Marfan's syndrome, Stickler's syndrome and Ehlers–Danlos syndrome.

Treatment modalities

The three modalities used for prophylaxis are: (a) cryotherapy, (b) laser photocoagulation using a slitlamp delivery system and (c) laser photocoagulation using the indirect ophthalmoscopic delivery system combined with scleral indentation. Most lesions can be adequately treated with either cryotherapy or laser photocoagulation. In most cases the treatment modality is based on the surgeon's preference and experience as well as the availability of instrumentation. Other considerations are as follows:

1. **Location of lesion**: an equatorial lesion can be treated by either photocoagulation or cryotherapy. A postequatorial lesion can be treated only by photocoagulation unless the conjuctiva is incised. Peripheral lesions near the ora serrata can be treated either by cryotherapy or laser photocoagulation using the indirect ophthalmoscope delivery system combined with indentation. Treatment of very peripheral lesions by laser photocoagulation using a slitlamp delivery system is difficult because it may be impossible to adequately treat the base of a U-tear.
2. **Clarity of media**: eyes with hazy media are much easier to treat by cryotherapy.
3. **Pupil size**: eyes with small pupils are easier to treat by cryotherapy.

Laser photocoagulation

Slitlamp delivery technique

1. Select a spot size of 200 μm and set the duration to 0.1 or 0.2 seconds.
2. Insert the triple-mirror contact lens or one of the wide field lenses.

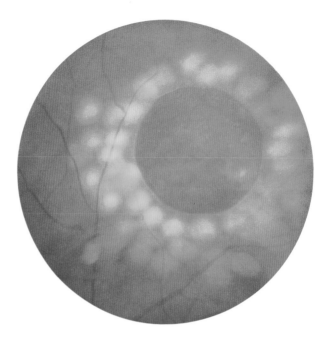

Figure 5.2 Appearance following prophylactic treatment of a large hole by argon laser photocoagulation

3. Surround the lesion with two rows of confluent burns of moderate intensity (Figure 5.2).
4. After treatment advise the patient to avoid strenuous physical exertion for about 7 days until an adequate adhesion has formed and the lesion is securely sealed.

Potential problems

Serious complications from peripheral retinal photocoagulation are rare. When they do occur, they are usually associated with excessively heavy treatment to large areas of the retina and may involve both anterior and posterior segments.

1. **Maculopathy** is in the form of cystoid macular oedema or macular pucker (Figure 5.3).
2. **Choroidal detachment**, which may be associated with secondary angle-closure glaucoma as a result of a forward rotation of the ciliary body.
3. **Exudative RD**, which usually resolves within 1 or 2 weeks.
4. **Rhegmatogenous RD** which is usually secondary to the formation of new retinal tears from excessively heavy treatment.
5. **Retinal haemorrhage** is rare and can usually be stopped by pressing the contact lens against the eye in order to increase intraocular pressure.
6. **Anterior segment** problems, which are rare, include: (a) corneal burns; (b) iris burns which may result in iritis, iris atrophy and sphincter damage; (c) anterior capsular lens opacities; and (d) transient myopia.

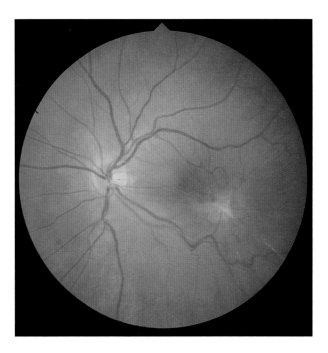

Figure 5.3 Macular pucker

Cryotherapy

Technique

1. Instil a topical anaesthetic. Some surgeons also inject ligno-caine (Xylocaine) subconjunctivally in the same quadrant as the lesion to be treated. For lesions behind the equator, a small conjunctival incision may be necessary to enable the cryoprobe to reach the required location.
2. Insert a Barraquer speculum.
3. Check the cryoprobe for correct freezing and defrosting and also make sure that the rubber sleeve is not covering the tip.
4. While viewing with the indirect ophthalmoscope, gently indent the sclera with the tip of the probe. In order not to mistake the shaft of the probe for the tip, start indenting near the ora serrata and then move the tip posteriorly to the lesion.
5. Surround the lesion with a single row of cryo-applications, terminating freezing as soon as the retina whitens. Because recently frozen retina soon reverts to its normal colour, it is easier to inadvertently re-treat the same area with cryother-apy than with photocoagulation.
6. Do not remove the cryoprobe until it has defrosted completely because premature removal may 'crack' the choroid and give rise to a choroidal haemorrhage.
7. Pad the eye for about 4 hours to prevent chemosis and advise the patient to refrain from strenuous physical activi-ties for 7 days.

71

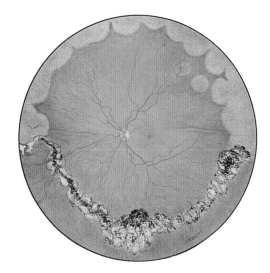

Figure 5.4 *Top:* oedema of the superior peripheral retina one day following prophylactic cryotherapy; *bottom:* pigmentation of the inferior peripheral retina four weeks following prophylactic cryotherapy

Postcryotherapy appearance

For about 2 days the treated area appears whitish due to oedema (Figure 5.4). After about 5 days pigmentation begins to appear. Initially the pigment is fine and then it becomes coarser and is associated with a variable amount of chorioretinal atrophy (Figure 5.5).

Potential problems

1. **Chemosis and lid oedema** are common and innocuous.
2. **Transient diplopia** may occur as a result of freezing of a rectus muscle.

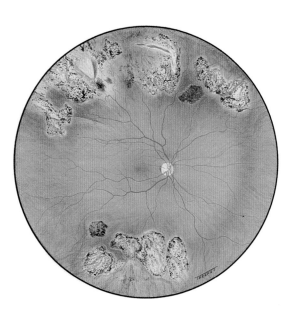

Figure 5.5 Moderate pigmentation and chorioretinal atrophy following prophylactic cryotherapy to retinal breaks and predisposing degenerations

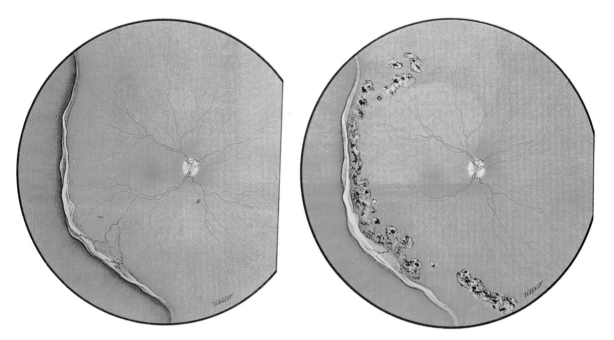

Figure 5.6 *Left:* giant traumatic dialysis before treatment; *right:* appearance following prophylactic cryotherapy – note that treatment is inadequate because the reaction is not continuous inferiorly and does not extend up to the ora serrata superiorly

3. **Vitritis** may occur as a result of excessively heavy treatment.
4. **Maculopathy** is very rare.

Causes of failure

The two main causes of failure of prophylaxis are: (a) inadequate treatment of the predisposing lesion and (b) the formation of new retinal breaks.

1. Failure to surround the entire lesion, particularly the base of a U-tear is the most common cause of failure. If the most peripheral part of the tear cannot be reached by photocoagulation then cryotherapy should be used.
2. Failure to apply contiguous treatment when treating a large break or a dialysis (Figure 5.6).
3. Failure to release dynamic vitreoretinal traction on a large U-tear by inserting an explant and failure to use an explant in an eye with a 'subclinical RD'.
4. New break formation (Figure 5.7) within or adjacent to treated area is usually caused by excessively heavy treatment, particularly of lattice degeneration. New break developing away from a treated area in apparently normal retina is probably unassociated with the treatment itself.

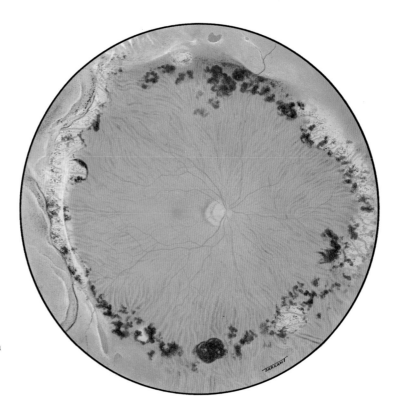

Figure 5.7 New retinal breaks at 12 o'clock and 7 o'clock with localized retinal detachment anterior to a barrage of prophylactic cryotherapy

Benign peripheral retinal degeneration

It is important to recognize the following entirely innocuous peripheral retinal degenerations (Figure 5.8) which do not require prophylaxis.

1. **Microcystoid degeneration** consists of tiny vesicles with indistinct boundaries on a greyish-white background which make the retina appear thickened and less transparent (Figure 5.8*a*). The degeneration always starts adjacent to the ora serrata and extends circumferentially and posteriorly with a smooth undulating posterior border. Microcystoid degeneration is present in all adult eyes, increasing in severity with age, and is not in itself causally related to RD, although it may give rise to retinoschisis.

2. **Snowflakes** are minute glistening yellow-white dots which are frequently found scattered diffusely in the peripheral fundus (Figure 5.8*b*). Occasionally, circumscribed aggregations of snowflakes may be seen near the equator. Foci composed solely of snowflakes are innocuous and require no treatment. Snowflakes are, however, of considerable clinical importance because, as already mentioned, they are

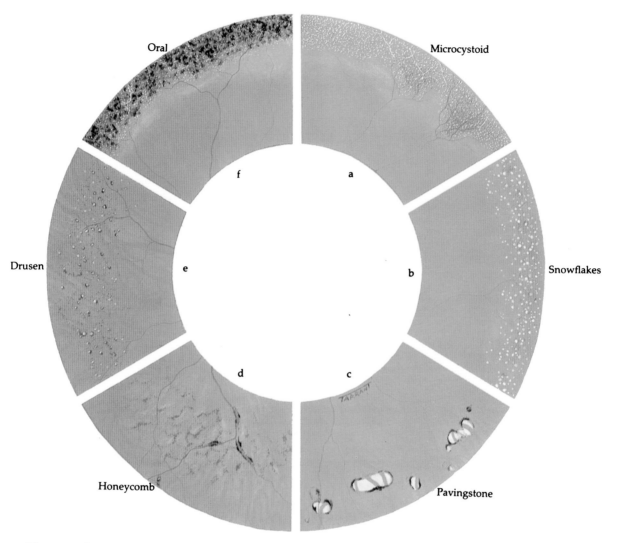

Figure 5.8 Benign peripheral retinal degenerations

frequently associated with lattice degeneration, snailtrack degeneration and acquired retinoschisis.

3. **Pavingstone degeneration** is characterized by discrete yellow-white patches of focal chorioretinal atrophy which is present to some extent in 25% of normal eyes (Figure 5.8c).

4. **Honeycomb (reticular) degeneration** is an age-related change characterized by a fine network of perivascular pigmentation which may extend posterior to the equator (Figure 5.8d).

5. **Drusen (colloid bodies)** are characterized by clusters of small pale lesions which may have hyperpigmented borders (Figure 5.8e). They are similar to drüsen at the posterior pole and usually occur in the eyes of elderly individuals.

6. **Oral pigmentary degeneration** is an age-related change consisting of a hyperpigmented band running adjacent to the ora serrata (Figure 5.8*f*).

Further reading

Aaberg, T. M. and Stevens, T. R. (1972) Snailtrack degeneration of the retina. *American Journal of Ophthalmology*, **73**, 370–376

Byer, N. E. (1974) Changes in and progression of lattice degeneration of the retina. *Transactions of the American Academy of Ophthalmology and Otolaryngology*, **78**, 114–125

Byer, N. E. (1986) Long-term natural history of senile retinoschisis with implications for management. *Ophthalmology*, **93**, 1127–1130

Byer, N. E. (1982) The natural history of asymptomatic retinal breaks. *Ophthalmology*, **89**, 1033–1039

Chignell, A. N. and Shilling, J. S. (1973) Prophylaxis of retinal detachment. *British Journal of Ophthalmology*, **57**, 291–298

Davis, M. D. (1974) Natural history of retinal breaks without detachment. *Archives of Ophthalmology*, **92**, 183–194

de Bustros, S. and Welch, R. B. (1984) The avulsed retinal vessel syndrome and its variants. *Ophthalmology*, **91**, 86–88

Folk, J. C., Arrindell, E. L. and Klugman, M. R. (1989) The fellow eye in patients with phakic lattice retinal detachments. *Ophthalmology*, **96**, 72–79

Kanski, J. J. (1975) Anterior segment complications of retinal photocoagulation. *American Journal of Ophthalmology*, **79**, 424–427

Kanski, J. J. and Daniel, R. (1975) Prophylaxis of retinal detachment. *American Journal of Ophthalmology*, **79**, 197–205

Lemesurier, R. and Chignell, A. H. (1981) Prophylaxis of aphakic retinal detachment. *Transactions of the Ophthalmological Society of the UK*, **101**, 212–213

McPherson, A., O'Malley, R. and Beltangady, S. S. (1981) Management of the fellow eye of patients with rhegmatogenous retinal detachment. *Ophthalmology*, **88**, 922–934

Morse, P. H. and Eagle, R. C. (1975) Pigmentation and retinal breaks. *American Journal of Ophthalmology*, **79**, 190–193

Pollak, A. and Oliver, M. (1981) Argon laser photocoagulation of symptomatic flap tears and retinal breaks of fellow eyes. *British Journal of Ophthalmology*, **65**, 469–472

Robertson, D. M. and Norton, E. W. D. (1973) Long term follow up of treated retinal breaks. *American Journal of Ophthalmology*, **75**, 395–404

Rutnin, U. and Schepens, C. L. (1967) Fundus appearance in normal eyes: III. Peripheral degenerations. *American Journal of Ophthalmology*, **64**, 1040-1062

Scott, J.D. (1989) Prevention and perspectives in retinal detachment. *Eye*, **3**, 491–515

6 Preoperative considerations

Prognosis for central vision

The two main factors governing eventual visual function, provided the retina has been successfully reattached, are: (a) duration of macular involvement and (b) extent of retinal elevation. If the macula is uninvolved most eyes maintain their preoperative visual acuity, although about 10% will develop impairment of central vision from some form of maculopathy (see Chapter 9). If the macula is involved for less than 2 months, most eyes have some impairment of central vision although, surprisingly, there appears to be no direct correlation between the duration of macular detachment and final visual acuity. Nevertheless, eyes with macular involvement should be operated on as soon as possible but not necessarily as emergencies. If the macula has been involved for over 2 months, postoperative visual acuity is usually very poor and its level is related to the duration of macular involvement. However, it must be emphasized that, although visual acuity may be poor, the patient is frequently glad to have restoration of peripheral vision. A less well documented prognostic factor is the amount of elevation of the detached retina at the posterior pole. It appears that the severity of photoreceptor cell degeneration in detached retina increases the greater its separation from the RPE.

Indications for urgent treatment

It should be noted that the spread of SRF is governed by three factors:

1. The position of the primary retinal break is important because SRF will spread more quickly if it is located superiorly.
2. The size of the break is also important because large breaks tend to lead to a more rapid accumulation of SRF than small ones.
3. State of vitreous gel; if the vitreous gel is healthy and solid, even giant retinal tears or giant dialyses (see Figure 5.6) may not lead to RD. However, if synchysis is advanced as in myopia, progression is usually rapid and the entire retina may become detached within 1 or 2 days.

It is therefore apparent that a patient with a fresh RD involving the superotemporal quadrant but with an intact macula (Figure 6.1) should be admitted immediately and operated on as soon as possible. In order to prevent SRF spreading to the macula, the patient should be positioned flat in bed with only one pillow and with the head turned so that the retinal break is in the most dependent position. For example, a patient with a right upper temporal RD should turn his head to the right. Preoperative bed rest is also desirable in eyes with bullous RDs (Figure 6.2) because it may lessen the amount of SRF which will facilitate the localization of retinal breaks during surgery, and may avoid the necessity to drain. Patients with fresh dense vitreous haemorrhage in whom visualization of the fundus is impossible should also be operated on as soon as possible if B-scan ultrasonography shows an underlying RD.

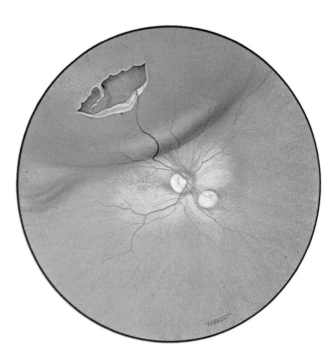

Figure 6.1 Fresh superior retinal detachment caused by a large retinal tear

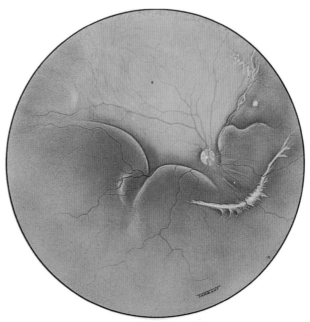

Figure 6.2 Bullous retinal detachment without a detectable break associated with a subretinal fibrous band

Problems associated with intraocular lens implants

1. Pupil dilatation may result in subluxation of an iris-supported lens.
2. Scleral indentation may be hazardous in eyes with rigid angle-supported lenses (Figure 6.3).
3. Lens reflexes may make slitlamp biomicroscopy difficult.
4. Capular opacification may impair visualization of the fundus (Figure 6.4).
5. Drainage of SRF eyes with rigid angle-supported lenses may distort the globe and cause bleeding from the chamber angle.
6. Intravitreal air injection may displace an iris-supported lens anteriorly and damage the corneal endothelium.

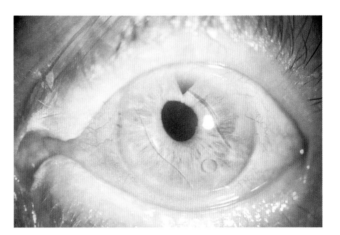

Figure 6.3 A rigid (Choyce) angle-supported intraocular implant

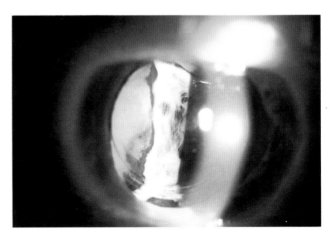

Figure 6.4 Severe capsular opacification

Mydriatics

Both eyes are dilated with 1% cyclopentolate and 10% phenylephrine drops given at 15-minute intervals for 2 hours preoperatively. One per cent atropine is also instilled into the eye to be operated in order to maintain good mydriasis postoperatively. In eyes with pupils that are difficult to dilate, a subconjunctival injection of Mydricaine (atropine, adrenaline and procaine) may be necessary.

Prophylactic antibiotics

Although postoperative intraocular infection is extremely rare following RD surgery, most surgeons use prophylactic antibiotics preoperatively. The most widely used antibiotic is gentamicin, which is instilled at 15-minute intervals for 2 hours prior to surgery. A solution of aqueous 5% povidone-iodine (Betadine) may also be used in the operating theatre immediately prior to surgery.

What to tell the patient

The function of the retina can be likened to the film in a camera and an RD can be explained in terms of wallpaper peeling off a wall. Simple diagrams may be helpful in explaining the principles of surgery. Inform the patient that the other eye will also be examined and any weaknesses will be treated by freezing. It is also important to emphasize that anatomical success does not equal visual success and occasionally a second operation is necessary. The patient should be warned that after surgery the eye will be red, tender and slightly painful. There may also be some transient double vision.

Further reading

Chisholm, I. A., McClure, E. and Foulds, W. S. (1975) Functional recovery of the retina after retinal detachment. *Transactions of the Ophthalmological Society of the UK*, **95**, 167–172

Davies, E. W. G. (1972) Factors affecting recovery of visual acuity following detachment. *Transactions of the Ophthalmological Society of the UK*, **92**, 335–344

Grupposo, S. S. (1975) Visual acuity following surgery for retinal detachment. *Archives of Ophthalmology*, **93**, 327–330

Lean, J. S., Mahmood, M., Manna, R. *et al.* (1980) Effect of preoperative posture and binocular occlusion on retinal detachment. *British Journal of Ophthalmology*, **64**, 94–97

Tani, P., Robertson, D. M. and Langworthy, A. (1981) A prognosis for central vision and anatomic reattachment in rhegmatogenous retinal detachment with macula detached. *American Journal of Ophthalmology*, **92**, 611–620

Wilkinson, C. P. (1981) Visual results following scleral buckling for retinal detachment sparing the macula. *Retina*, **1**, 113–116

Wilkinson, C.P. (1985) Pseudophakic retinal detachments. *Retina*, **5**, 1–4

7 Principles of standard retinal surgery

General considerations

Local explants
General properties
Indications

Encircling explants
General properties
Indications

Drainage of subretinal fluid
Indications
Advantages of drainage

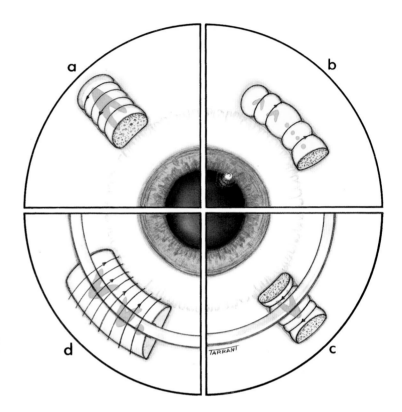

Figure 7.1 Configuration of scleral buckles. (*a*), Radial sponge explant; (*b*), circumferential sponge explant; (*c*), encirclement augmented by a radial sponge explant; (*d*), encirclement augmented by a solid silicone tyre

General considerations

Scleral buckling is a surgical procedure for creating an inward indentation of the sclera ('buckle'). Its two main purposes are: (a) to close retinal breaks by apposing the RPE to the sensory retina and (b) to reduce dynamic vitreoretinal traction at sites of local vitreoretinal adhesion. An explant is material sutured directly onto the sclera to create a buckle. It may have one of the following configurations:

1. **Radial** explants are placed at right angles to the limbus (Figure 7.1*a*).
2. **Segmental circumferential** explants are placed circumferentially with the limbus to create a segmental buckle (Figure 7.1*b*).
3. **Encircling** explants are placed around the entire circumference of the globe to create a 360° buckle (Figure 7.1*c* and *d*).

All explants are made from either soft or hard silicone as follows:

1. **Soft silicone (Silastic) sponges** may be round or oval. Round sponges have a diameter of 3 mm, 4 mm and 5 mm, and oval sponges are 5.5 × 7.5 mm. Sponges are most

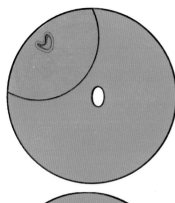

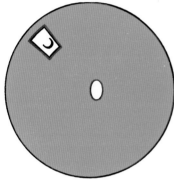

Figure 7.2 Treatment of a retinal detachment associated with a solitary U-tear (*top*) by a radial buckle (*bottom*)

frequently used for local buckling and may also be used to supplement an encircling strap (Figure 7.1*c*). Occasionally, they are also used for encirclement.

2. **Hard silicone straps** are used only for 360° buckling.
3. **Hard silicone tyres** of various dimensions may be used either to create solitary local buckles or to supplement an encircling strap (Figure 7.1*d*).

Local explants

General properties

In order to adequately seal a retinal break it is essential for the buckle to have adequate length, width and height. The entire break should be surrounded by about 2 mm of buckle. It is also important for the buckle to involve the area of the vitreous base anterior to the tear in order to prevent the possibility of subsequent reopening of the tear and anterior leakage of SRF. The dimensions of the retinal break are assessed by comparing it with the diameter of the optic disc (1.5 mm).

1. The width of a *radial buckle* depends on the width (distance between anterior horns) of the retinal tear and its length depends on the length (distance between base and apex) of the tear. In general, the width of the explant should be twice that of the tear.
2. The width of a *segmental circumferential buckle* depends on the length of the tear and the length of the buckle depends on the width of the tear.

The eventual height of a local buckle is determined by the following interrelated factors.

1. The greater the diameter of the explant, the higher the buckle. Cutting a sponge in half lengthways will reduce its circumference without affecting its diameter.
2. The greater the separation of sutures, the higher the buckle.
3. The tighter the sutures over the explant, the higher the buckle.
4. The lower the intraocular pressure, the higher the buckle. However, if the eye is rock hard it will be impossible to create a buckle irrespective of the diameter of the explant, separation of sutures and tightness of sutures. Conversely, in a very soft eye, a high buckle can be created with a small-diameter sponge. Most local buckles lose their effect after about 3 years.

Indications

Radial buckling

1. Large U-tears, because there is less tendency to 'fishmouthing' (Figure 7.2).

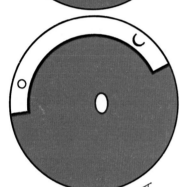

Figure 7.3 Treatment of a retinal detachment associated with two breaks in different quadrants (*top*) by a circumferential buckle (*bottom*)

2. Relatively posterior breaks, because sutures are easier to insert.

Segmental circumferential buckling

1. Multiple breaks located in one or two quadrants and/or at varying distances from the ora serrata (Figure 7.3).
2. Anterior breaks because they can be closed more easily.
3. Wide breaks such as dialyses (see Figure 4.6).

A solitary hole can be sealed with either a radial or a circumferential buckle.

Encircling explants

General properties

1. Straps are most frequently used for encirclement. The most commonly used has a diameter of 2 mm (no. 40) although wider straps are available. A strap induces a fairly narrow buckle which frequently has to be supplemented with either radial sponges or circumferential solid silicone tyres to support large tears. A 2 mm high buckle can be produced by shortening the strap by about 12 mm. In contrast to a local explant, the buckle produced by a strap is permanent.
2. Encirclement with a 3 mm or 4 mm sponge gives a broader buckle than a strap and may obviate the necessity to place additional radial explants.

Indications

1. Breaks involving three or more quadrants.
2. Lattice or snailtrack degeneration involving three or more quadrants (Figure 7.4).
3. Extensive RD without detectable breaks, particularly in eyes with hazy media, intraocular lens implants or aphakia. A broad buckle is used in an attempt to seal breaks anterior to the equator.
4. Moderate PVR to create a permanent 360° buckle by reducing the diameter of the globe at the equator.
5. Failed local procedures in which the reason for failure is not apparent.

Drainage of subretinal fluid

Indications

Although a large proportion of RDs can be treated successfully with non-drainage techniques, drainage of SRF may be required under the following circumstances:

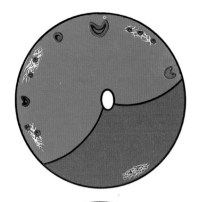

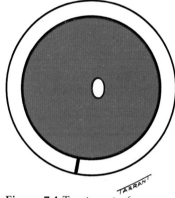

Figure 7.4 Treatment of a retinal detachment associated with breaks and lattice degeneration involving several quadrants (*top*) by an encirclement (*bottom*)

1. **Difficulty in localization** of retinal breaks in bullous and highly elevated retina, particularly if the breaks are located behind the equator, is a relatively common indication. In such situations, air can be injected into the vitreous cavity to reconstitute normal intraocular pressure and to provide internal tamponade of the retinal break.

2. **Immobile retina** is an indication for drainage because the non-drainage procedure is successful only if the detached retina is sufficiently mobile to move back against the buckle during the postoperative period. If it is rendered relatively immobile by PVR, a high buckle is required to seal the break. This can be achieved only if the eye is first softened by draining the SRF.

3. **Long-standing RDs** tend to be associated with viscous SRF and may take a long time (many months) to absorb. Drainage may therefore be necessary, even if the break can be closed without drainage.

4. **Inferior RDs** associated with equatorial tears should probably be drained because, when the patient assumes the upright position postoperatively, any residual SRF will gravitate inferiorly and may reopen the tear. Most dialyses, however, can be closed without drainage.

5. **Danger from raised intraocular pressure**: eyes in which significant elevation of intraocular pressure may cause problems should be drained. This is because with a non-drainage procedure the scleral sutures have to be tightened over the sponge in order to achieve the desired buckling effect. This causes a significant elevation of intraocular pressure for several hours. As the pressure gradient is reduced, the sponge expands inwards and closes the retinal tear. After the tear is closed, any residual SRF usually absorbs within 24–48 hours. The temporary elevation of intraocular pressure is usually harmless although in the following situations it may have detrimental effects:
    (a) In eyes with advanced glaucomatous field loss it may cause a complete loss of all vision.
    (b) In eyes with thin sclera the sutures may cut out as they are being tightened.
    (c) In eyes which have undergone cataract extraction within the last 6 weeks because the incision may rupture.

Advantages of drainage

Although non-drainage of SRF avoids most of the operative complications, which will be described in the following chapter, drainage provides immediate contact between the sensory retina and RPE with flattening of the fovea. If this contact is delayed for more than 5 days, a satisfactory adhesion will not develop around the retinal break because the 'stickiness' of the RPE will have worn off. This may result in non-attachment of the retina or, in some cases, reopening of the break during the postoperative period. In addition, drainage of SRF allows the use of a large bubble of an internal tamponading agent (air or gas).

Further reading

Goldbaum, M. H., Smithline, M., Poole, A. *et al.* (1975) Geometric analysis of radial buckles. *American Journal of Ophthalmology*, **79**, 958–965
Lincoff, H. A. and Kreissig, I. (1975) Advantages of radial buckles. *American Journal of Ophthalmology*, **79**, 955–957

8   # Techniques of standard retinal surgery

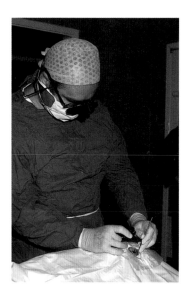

Figure 8.1 Preliminary examination of the fundus using scleral indentation

Preoperative preparation

1. Both pupils should be widely dilated and the eyelids of the fellow eye taped shut to prevent corneal exposure.
2. Two drops of 5% povidone-iodine solution should be instilled into the conjunctival sac and the lids gently manipulated to distribute it evenly over the ocular surface. The solution is made up by diluting the full-strength 10% Betadine aqueous solution used for skin preparation with 1:1 balanced saline.
3. One person should be assigned to operate the lights.
4. The retinal drawing should be displayed upside down in a convenient place.
5. Before mounting the indirect ophthalmoscope make sure the battery is fully charged and a spare is readily available.
6. Prep the skin but make sure that it has been dried because Steridrape will not adhere to wet skin.
7. Insert a Barraquer speculum; it is preferred to the more bulky Lang's.
8. Irrigate the povidone-iodine from the conjunctival sac. Use a decent-sized cannula so that irrigation is quick and thorough. Bottles containing balanced salt solution (BSS) are better than syringes as they do not need to be refilled and can be quickly exchanged when empty.

Fundus examination

Perform a careful examination of the entire fundus using scleral indentation (Figure 8.1) and compare the findings with the fundus drawing:

1. Remind yourself of the location of breaks and predisposing degenerations.
2. Check that all important lesions are correctly indicated in the fundus drawing.
3. Note any changes in location or volume of SRF.
4. Assess retinal mobility by moving the eye with a squint hook; good retinal mobility, manifested by a free undulating movement of the detached retina, signifies absence of significant PVR.
5. Try to appose the retinal break to the RPE by indenting the sclera with a squint hook; if achieved easily, drainage of SRF may not be necessary.
6. Assess the dimensions of retinal breaks by comparison with the diameter of the optic nerve (1.5 mm). Remember that a retinal break in highly elevated retina appears larger and more posterior and therefore more difficult to manage than one of the same size in a shallow RD.

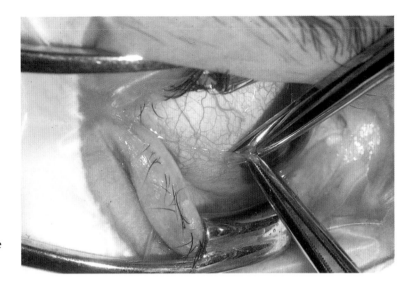

Figure 8.2 Initial incision of the conjunctiva and Tenon's capsule at the limbus

Exposure of the operative field

Peritomy

1. Pick up conjunctiva and Tenon's capsule near the limbus with Moorfields forceps and, with blunt-ended scissors, cut down to sclera (Figure 8.2). Because conjunctiva and Tenon's capsule are fused at the limbus, both will be incised together.
2. With scissors, undermine conjunctiva and Tenon's and cut circumferentially with the limbus (Figure 8.3). The least extent of peritomy is about 100°, to include two rectus muscles, and greatest is 360° to expose four recti.

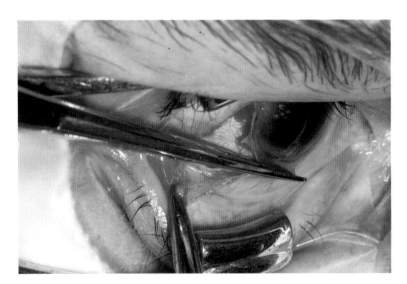

Figure 8.3 Circumferential incision around the limbus

3. Grasp the cut end of the conjunctiva with forceps and lift it away from the sclera.
4. Slide closed scissors posteriorly over the sclera and break the episclera-Tenon's adhesion by opening the blades; take care not to tear the conjunctiva or damage vortex veins.
5. Make relaxing 6 mm incisions at right angles with the limbus; take care not to damage the plica semilunaris nasally.
6. With cellulose sponges, clear the episcleral tissue from the sclera to facilitate subsequent insertion of scleral sutures and drainage of SRF; beginners frequently do not appreciate the importance of this step.
7. Cut the check ligaments of the exposed muscles. If reoperating, previously inserted buckling material may have to be removed.

Insertion of bridle sutures

Bridle sutures are used to stabilize the globe and manipulate it into optimal positions during surgery. The technique is as follows:

1. Insert a squint hook under a rectus muscle (Figure 8.4); if working under the superior rectus make sure you have separated it from the underlying superior oblique.
2. Pass a reverse mounted needle with a 4/0 black silk suture under (not through) the muscle tendon (Figure 8.5).
3. Secure the suture by twisting it around mosquito forceps (Figure 8.6) and cut off the excess.
4. Repeat steps 1–3 for other tendons as required.

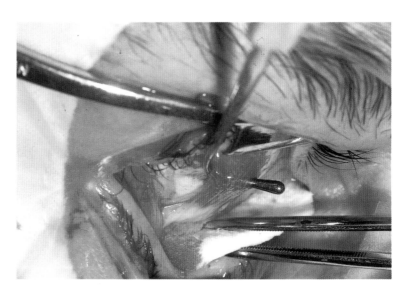

Figure 8.4 Insertion of a squint hook under a rectus muscle

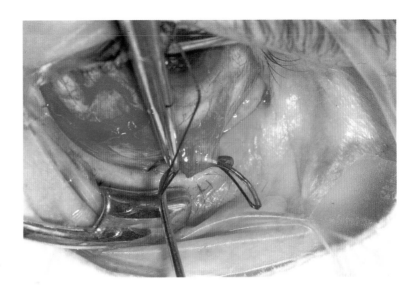

Figure 8.5 Insertion of a bridle suture under a rectus muscle

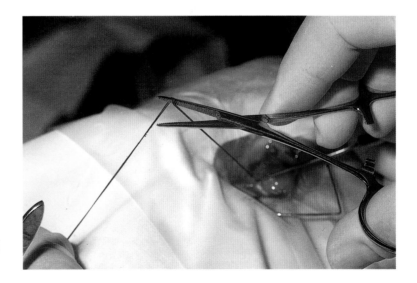

Figure 8.6 Twisting of the bridle suture around mosquito forceps

Inspection of the sclera

The purpose of scleral inspection is two-fold.

1. **To detect anomalous vortex veins** so that they will not be damaged during cryotherapy, scleral buckling or drainage of SRF.
2. **To detect scleral thinning** (Figure 8.7) which may be associated with the following problems:
   (a) Penetration of the choroid and retina during insertion of scleral sutures.

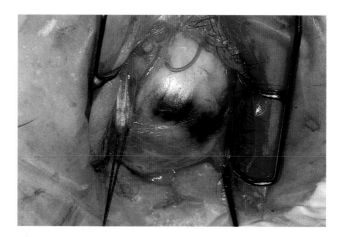

Figure 8.7 Severe scleral thinning

(b) Cutting out of sutures as they are being tightened over the explant. This is particularly likely to occur when the intraocular pressure is elevated because SRF has not been drained.
(c) Scleral rupture during cryotherapy or localization of breaks.

Localization of breaks

Technique

The purpose of localization is to place the buckle in the correct position. The technique is as follows:

1. Insert a 5/0 Dacron scleral suture at the site calculated to correspond to the apex of the tear; take care not to insert the needle too deeply as this may result in premature release of SRF. Remember that most breaks are located near the equator, which is 12–13 mm behind the limbus in an emmetropic eye. Also try to avoid the tendency to localize breaks too posteriorly in eyes with deep SRF.
2. Tie the suture with a double throw and trim to 1 cm.
3. Grasp the cut suture with curved mosquito forceps as close to the knot as possible (Figure 8.8).
4. While viewing with the indirect ophthalmoscope, indent the sclera by rotating the forceps away from the globe.
5. If the indentation does not coincide with the break, repeat the procedure until accurate localization is achieved (Figure 8.9). In eyes with very large breaks such as dialyses or giant tears, localize the two ends as well as the midpoint of the posterior flap. Long islands of lattice degeneration should also be localized if they are to be included in the buckle.

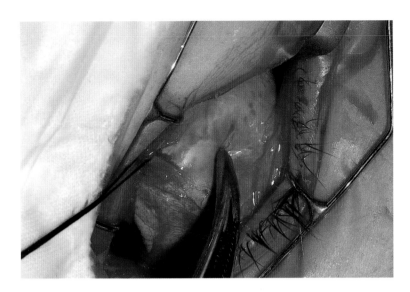

Figure 8.8 Base of localizing suture grasped with mosquito forceps

An alternative method of localization is to use a special scleral depressor which will leave a circular mark on the sclera when pressed vertically. Because the mark is temporary it is necessary to make a permanent mark with either a methylene-blue marker, gentle cautery or diathermy.

Potential problems

Localization of relatively anterior breaks in eyes with shallow SRF is easy. However, accurate localization may be very difficult

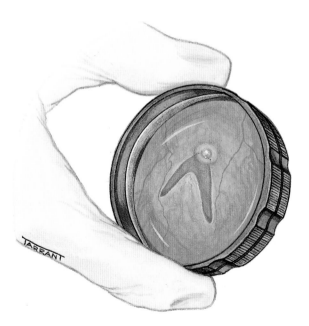

Figure 8.9 Accurate localization of the apex of a large U-tear

or impossible in eyes with bullous RDs, especially if associated with breaks located behind the equator. In these cases adequate localization can be achieved by using the D-ACE (Drain-Air-Cryo-Explant) technique as follows:

1. Drain the SRF to bring the break closer to the RPE.
2. Inject air into the vitreous cavity to counteract the hypotony induced by drainage.
3. Localize the break and apply cryotherapy.
4. Insert the explant.

Cryotherapy

Technique

Cryotherapy creates an inflammatory chorioretinal lesion which, on scarring, results in a stronger than normal bond between the sensory retina and RPE so that retinal breaks are permanently sealed. The technique is as follows:

1. Check that the cryoprobe is able to freeze to −80°C and defrost quickly.
2. Ask the assistant to stabilize the globe with traction sutures.
3. Ask for the theatre lights to be turned off.
4. Ask the assistant not to irrigate the cornea during freezing.
5. Indent the sclera gently with the tip of the cryoprobe while viewing with the indirect ophthalmoscope (Figure 8.10).
6. Commence freezing by depressing the footswitch and continue until the sensory retina has just turned white (Figure 8.11).

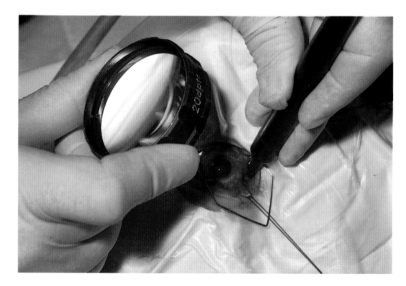

Figure 8.10 Cryotherapy

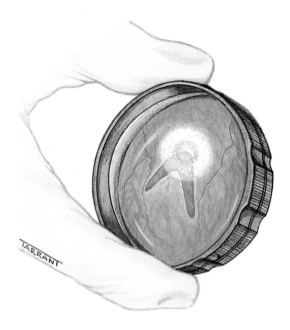

Figure 8.11 Cryotherapy causing whitening of the sensory retina

7. First treat any predisposing lesions in attached retina as this will soften the globe and may facilitate subsequent treatment of breaks in detached retina.
8. When freezing breaks in detached retina, indent the sclera with the cryoprobe to bring the RPE as close as possible to the break. The break will appear darker as a result of the contrast between the white frozen sensory retina and the underlying RPE and choroid. This phenomenon is useful in differentiating small breaks from areas of retinal thinning.
9. Repeat cryotherapy until the entire break has been surrounded by a 2 mm margin. Small holes may require only one application whereas large tears or long islands of lattice degeneration will require several.
10. Secure the cryoprobe to the instrument trolley so it will not fall off.

Potential problems

Failure of iceball to appear

If after about 6 seconds the iceball cannot be visualized, check the following:

1. Make sure that you are not mistaking the shaft of the probe for the tip and are not freezing the macula.
2. Check that the probe is freezing to $-80\,°C$.
3. Make sure that you are not trying to freeze through the patient's eyelids or through a rectus muscle.

97

Excessive cryotherapy

Excessive freezing is undesirable because it predisposes to pigment fallout, postoperative vitritis and exudative RD (see Chapter 9). It can be prevented by taking the following precautions:

1. Avoid refreezing the same area several times. If cryotherapy has to be applied to a large area, refreezing can be avoided by observing normal anatomical landmarks and also noting that recently frozen retina becomes less transparent after about 30 seconds.
2. In eyes with very deep SRF it may be impossible to freeze the sensory retina without the formation of a huge iceball within the subretinal space. In these circumstances it may be necessary to perform the D-ACE procedure to ensure that both the RPE and sensory retina are adequately treated.

Insufficient cryotherapy

Insufficient cryotherapy is undesirable because it may result in redetachment of the retina. The following are the main reasons:

1. Failure to correctly detect the end-point due to hazy media or deep SRF.
2. Malfunction of the cryoprobe.
3. Malposition of the cryoprobe.

Miscellaneous problems

1. Premature removal of the cryoprobe should be resisted because 'cracking' the tip of the probe off the sclera before the iceball has defrosted may cause: (a) choroidal haemorrhage by 'cracking' the frozen choroid and (b) rupture of thin sclera.
2. Excessive indentation of the sclera with the cryoprobe, in vulnerable eyes, may result in the following: (a) intraocular penetration through thin sclera, (b) rupture of a cataract incision and (c) closure of the central retinal artery.

Scleral buckling techniques

The instruments required for scleral buckling are: (a) two Castroviejo needleholders, (b) calipers, (c) retractor, (d) cautery and (e) 5/0 Dacron double-ended sutures on a spatulated needle; a quarter-circle needle is best for long anterior placement but a half-circle needle is preferred for relatively posterior placement.

Local explants

1. Select the appropriate-sized explant according to the criteria described in Chapter 7. The explant may be either a solid silicone tyre or Silastic sponge.

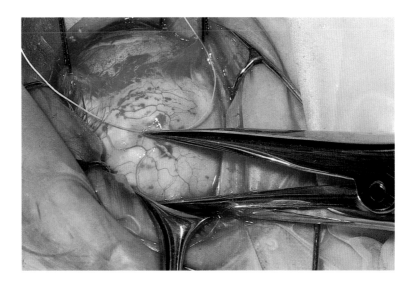

Figure 8.12 Measurement of separation of the sutures

2. With calipers, measure the distance separating the sutures (Figure 8.12) and mark the sclera with cautery. As a general rule, the separation of sutures should be about 1.5× the diameter of the explant. For example, with a 4 mm explant separation of sutures should be 6 mm (i.e. 4 + 2), and for a 5 mm explant 7.5 mm (i.e. 5 + 2.5). If a very high buckle is desired, space the sutures even further apart.

3. Insert a mattress-type suture which will straddle the explant (Figure 8.13). The number of sutures will depend upon the length of the explant. Each bite should extend for about 5 mm and have an even intrascleral course. For radial buckles the tip of the needle should be pointing posteriorly as it traverses the sclera.

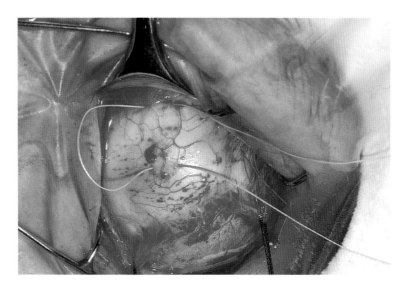

Figure 8.13 Insertion of mattress sutures

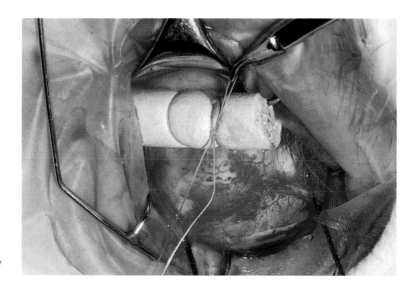

Figure 8.14 Tying of temporary bow

4. Pick up one end of the explant with the mosquito forceps and feed it through the sutures.
5. With two Castroviejo needleholders, tighten the sutures over the explant with a triple throw and then tie a temporary bow (Figure 8.14).
6. Check the position of the buckle in relation to the retinal break with the indirect ophthalmoscope and take appropriate action as follows:
   (a) If the break is closed or very nearly closed and there are no other open breaks, the operation can be terminated without drainage of SRF. Remember that the anterior extent of the buckle should include the area of the vitreous base.
   (b) If the buckle is incorrectly positioned it should be removed and repositioned.
   (c) If the position of the buckle is uncertain because of bullous elevation of the retina, SRF should be drained to ensure correct positioning.
7. Check the central retinal artery by inspecting the optic disc. If spontaneous pulsation is present, the intraocular pressure is between diastolic and systolic blood pressures and no specific action is required. If spontaneous pulsation is absent, the intraocular pressure is either below diastolic or above systolic. In this situation exert pressure on the globe with a squint hook and observe the disc.
   (a) If pulsation is induced, intraocular pressure is below diastolic (this is usually quite obvious anyway).
   (b) If pulsation is not induced, intraocular pressure is above systolic. In this event slacken the sutures and massage the globe for 2 minutes and then tighten the sutures very

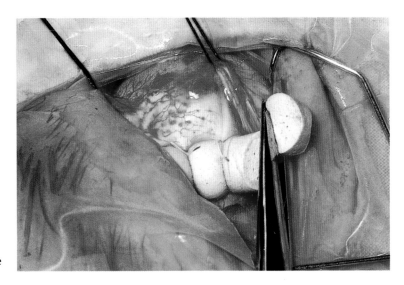

Figure 8.15 Trimming of sponge

slowly. If the central retinal artery is still occluded then either drain the SRF or perform a paracentesis of the anterior chamber.

8. Ask the assistant to stretch the sponge by pulling on the two ends with the mosquito forceps.
9. Convert the temporary bow into a permanent knot by utilizing two single throws.
10. Trim the edges of the sponge (Figure 8.15) so that they will not erode through the conjunctiva postoperatively.

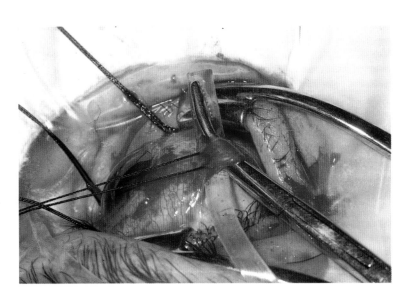

Figure 8.16 Sliding of the end of a strap under a rectus muscle

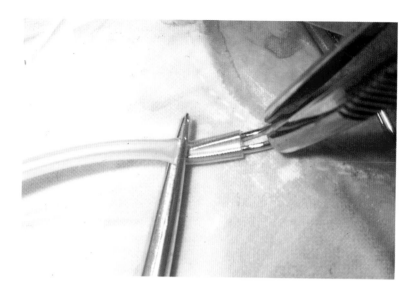

Figure 8.17 Preparation of the Watzke sleeve

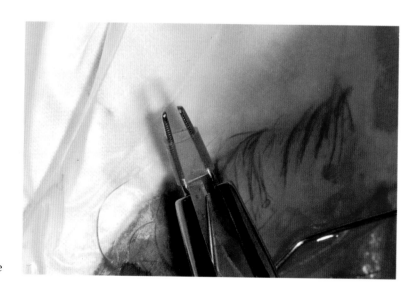

Figure 8.18 End of strap being inserted into the Watzke sleeve

Encircling procedures

1. Select the strap of appropriate diameter.
2. Grasp one end of the strap with curved mosquito forceps and feed it under the four recti (Figure 8.16), making sure that it does not become twisted.
3. Secure the two ends with a Watzke sleeve as follows:
   (a) Slide the sleeve (silicone tubing) over the ends of Watzke sleeve-spreading forceps and cut off about 5 mm (Figure 8.17).

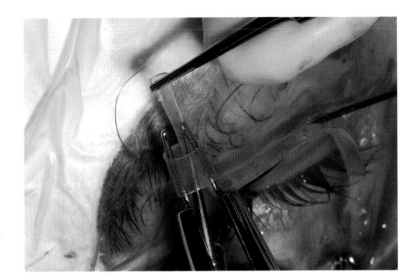

Figure 8.19 End of strap being pulled through the Watzke sleeve

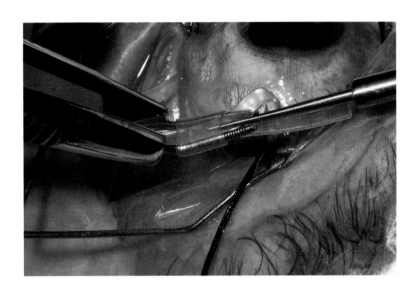

Figure 8.20 Other end of strap being pulled through the Watzke sleeve

(b) Grasp one end of the strap with forceps, stretch the sleeve with the Watzke forceps and pass the strap through the sleeve (Figure 8.18).

(c) Grip the end of the strap and pull it through the sleeve (Figure 8.19).

(d) Grasp the other end of the strap and push it through the sleeve above the strap already in place (Figure 8.20).

(e) Pull the strap through the sleeve and withdraw the forceps.

(f) Push the sleeve off the Watzke forceps (Figure 8.21).

103

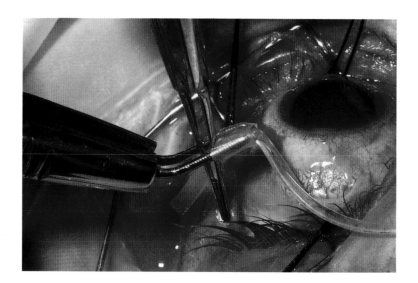

Figure 8.21 Disengagement of the Watzke sleeve

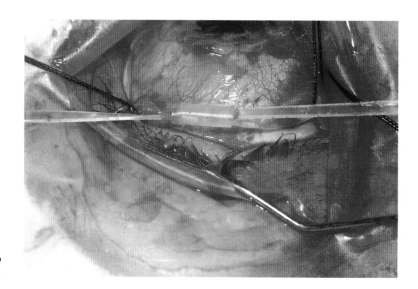

Figure 8.22 Tightening of strap with Watzke sleeve in position

4. Tighten the strap by pulling on the two ends (Figure 8.22) until it fits snugly around the ora serrata (Figure 8.23) and trim the ends.
5. Slide the strap posteriorly (about 4 mm) (Figure 8.24) and secure it in each quadrant with a holding suture (Figure 8.25). Take relatively small bites in the sclera and do not excessively tighten the sutures over the strap because their only purpose is to prevent the strap from sliding anteriorly or posteriorly.

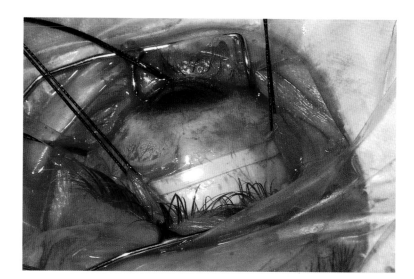

Figure 8.23 Encircling band fitting snugly but not too tightly around the ora serrata

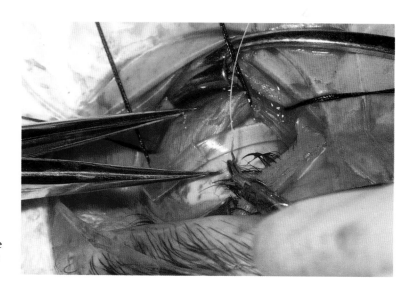

Figure 8.24 Measurement of the distance from the limbus to the eventual position of the strap

6. Tighten the strap to produce the required amount of internal indentation (Figure 8.26) as observed with the indirect ophthalmoscopy. An ideal height is about 2 mm which can be achieved by shortening the circumference of the strap by about 12 mm.
7. If necessary, insert under one part of the strap either a radial sponge, to support a large U-tear, or a circumferential tyre to support several breaks making sure that the anterior extension of the buckle involves the area of the vitreous base.

105

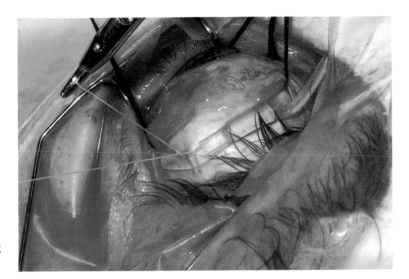

Figure 8.25 Insertion of holding suture

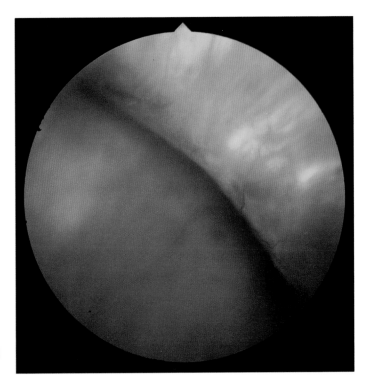

Figure 8.26 Indentation induced by an encircling strap

Potential problems

Accidental drainage of SRF

Accidental drainage of SRF may become apparent immediately or when the sutures are being tightened over the sponge, at

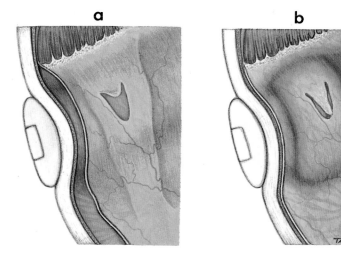

Figure 8.27 (*a*), 'fishmouthing' of a U-tear communicating with a radial retinal fold; (*b*), correction of 'fishmouthing' by insertion of an additional radial buckle

which point the SRF begins to leak out and the eye becomes soft. Premature drainage of SRF is undesirable because the induced ocular hypotony makes further suture placement difficult. Management depends on whether or not planned drainage was being contemplated as follows:

1. If drainage was contemplated, remove the offending suture and allow drainage to continue.
2. If drainage was not contemplated, quickly try to oversew the perforation and seal the drainage site. This may be difficult because the eye may become soft very rapidly so that intravitreal air injection may be necessary to restore the intraocular pressure to an acceptable level.

'Fishmouthing' phenomenon

'Fishmouthing' is a tendency of certain retinal tears, typically large superior U-tears located at the equator in a bullous RD, to open widely following scleral buckling and drainage of SRF. In some cases the RD may even appear more elevated than before and associated radial folds (Figure 8.27*a*) may make the tear very difficult to close. This may result in failure or delay in reattachment of the retina. Management of 'fishmouthing' is as follows:

1. Add extra radially orientated buckling material (Figure 8.27*b*).
2. Inject air into the vitreous cavity and position the patient postoperatively so that the bubble is closing the tear.

Radial retinal folds

Radial retinal folds may occasionally form as the retina drapes over the buckle. This problem usually occurs either when relatively long and posteriorly located circumferential buckles

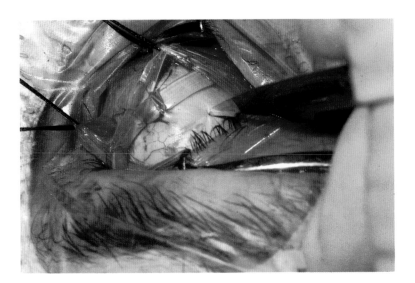

Figure 8.28 Radial sclerotomy for draining subretinal fluid

are used or when an encircling buckle is tied too tightly. Some folds flatten spontaneously during the postoperative period whilst others prevent retinal reattachment by keeping open a communicating retinal break. Management is as follows:

1. If the encircling element is too tight, loosen it.
2. Injection of air into the vitreous cavity will flatten most folds.
3. If the folds persist postoperatively and prevent retinal reattachment they can sometimes be flattened by applying photocoagulation around the break in the hope that the additional swelling so created will close the break and flatten the fold.

Miscellaneous

1. **Occlusion of central retinal artery** can be prevented by inspecting the central retinal artery after the sutures have been tightened as already described.
2. **Iatrogenic break formation** is a serious complication which may be associated with vitreous prolapse. The cause is an excessively deep placement of a suture, particularly in thin sclera. Management is as follows: (a) excise the prolapsed vitreous (if present) and (b) apply cryotherapy to the retinal tear and try to cover it with the buckle.

Drainage of subretinal fluid

Technique

1. Examine the fundus to make sure that the SRF has not shifted.

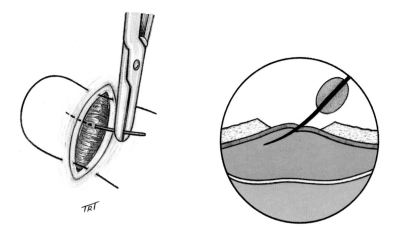

Figure 8.29 Technique of drainage of subretinal fluid with a suture needle

2. Make sure that the intraocular pressure is not elevated by relaxing the traction sutures and lifting the lid speculum from the globe. Drainage of SRF when the intraocular pressure is high may cause retinal incarceration.
3. Choose the sclerotomy site (see later).
4. Perform a radial sclerotomy about 4 mm long (Figure 8.28) of sufficient depth to allow herniation of a small dark knuckle of choroid into the incision.
5. Place a 5/0 Dacron mattress suture across the lips of the sclerotomy (optional).
6. Ask the assistant to hold the lips of the sclerotomy apart and inspect the prolapsed knuckle with a +20D lens for the presence of large choroidal vessels. These are usually obvious as they are located most superficially in the choroid. Large choroidal vessels can also be detected by transillumination through the pupil with a special fibreoptic light; the light from an indirect ophthalmoscope is inadequate.
7. If a large vessel is present, suture the sclerotomy and choose another drainage site.
8. If large choroidal vessels are absent, gently apply low heat cautery to the choroidal knuckle to prevent the possibility of choroidal bleeding; do not worry if this results in release of SRF.
9. If SRF has not been released, perforate the choroidal knuckle with one of the following:
   (a) A 25-gauge hypodermic needle on a syringe.
   (b) A sharp suture needle held by a needleholder (Figure 8.29).
   (c) Diathermy pin.
   (d) Argon endolaser probe.
   A sharp-ended instrument should be introduced tangentially to reduce the risk of retinal damage.
10. It is not always advantageous to drain all the SRF because the eye may become excessively soft. If necessary, partial

drainage can be performed by tying the sclerotomy suture into a temporary bow before all the SRF has been drained. The fundus can then be inspected and, if the tear is well placed on the buckle, the bow can be converted into a permanent knot. This partial drainage of SRF may obviate the necessity to perform an intravitreal injection to counter-act excessive ocular hypotony due to drainage of a large volume of SRF.

11. While the SRF is draining, gradually tighten the sutures over the buckling material to prevent hypotony.
12. Inspect the sclerotomy: the presence of small pigment granules means that all the SRF has been drained but do not mistake the viscous yellowish SRF in eyes with long-standing RDs for vitreous.
13. Inspect the fundus to check that the tear is correctly positioned on the buckle (as previously described) and to ensure that the retina is not incarcerated; a normal drainage site is apparent as a small yellow spot.
14. Knot the sclerotomy if a suture has been used.

Potential problems

Choroidal haemorrhage

Choroidal haemorrhage is usually caused by damaging a large choroidal vessel. Although small bleeds may be innocuous because the blood escapes with the SRF, large bleeds may give rise to the following complications.

1. Postoperative maculopathy and impairment of central vision may occur as a result of gravitation of large amounts of blood in the subretinal space to the fovea (see Chapter 9).
2. Vitreous haemorrhage as a result of entry of blood into the vitreous cavity through the retinal break.
3. Haemorrhagic choroidal detachment resulting from collection of a large volume of blood in the suprachoroidal space.

Prevention
1. Avoid drainage near the vortex ampullae; drainage is usually safe under or just on either side of the vertical recti anterior to the equator as well as just above and below (but not under) the horizontal recti.
2. Avoid drainage through recently frozen sclera because cryotherapy dilates choroidal vessels and increases the risk of bleeding.
3. Avoid drainage, if possible, in the temporal fundus because in the event of bleeding into the subretinal space the blood may not gravitate towards the fovea.

Management
Management of significant choroidal haemorrhage is as follows:

1. Tighten the sutures over the buckle as quickly as possible in order to increase intraocular pressure and prevent further bleeding.
2. Prevent gravitation of blood in the subretinal space to the fovea by rotating the globe and turning the patient's head.

Drainage of suprachoroidal blood by performing a second sclerotomy is unrewarding because the blood has already clotted.

Ocular hypotony

A sudden prolonged period of severe ocular hypotony is undesirable as it may lead to the following complications:

1. Choroidal haemorrhage due to rupture of a large choroidal vessel usually occurs away from the drainage site after SRF has been drained. Highly myopic eyes in which there has been a rapid drop of intraocular pressure are said to be at particular risk.
2. Miosis.
3. Postoperative choroidal detachment (see Chapter 9).
4. Hyphaema in eyes with rigid angle-supported intraocular lenses.

Prevention
1. Avoid a rapid evacuation of large amounts of SRF.
2. Avoid a prolonged period of severe hypotony by gradually tightening the sutures over the buckling material while the SRF is draining. Very occasionally, intravitreal injections are necessary to counteract severe hypotony (see later).

Dry tap

Failure of drainage of SRF (dry tap) may be caused by one of the following:

1. Failure to perforate the full thickness of the choroid.
2. Attempted drainage in an area of flat retina: therefore always check the position of the SRF immediately prior to drainage.
3. Incarceration of the retina in the sclerotomy (see later).

Iatrogenic break formation

An iatrogenic break is caused by perforation of the retina with the needle while draining SRF.

Prevention
1. Do not insert the needle too deeply into the subretinal space.
2. Drain where the SRF is deepest – usually near the equator.

3. Before draining, check the following:
   (a) There is still sufficient SRF to drain.
   (b) The SRF has not shifted.

Management
1. If retinal perforation has occurred within the bed of the buckle, no further action is necessary provided adequate cryotherapy has been applied to the area of the iatrogenic break.
2. Retinal perforation outside the bed of the buckle is managed as follows:
   (a) If the break is in detached retina, apply cryotherapy to the break and mount it on a small explant.
   (b) If the break is in flat retina, apply cryotherapy only.

Retinal incarceration

Incarceration of the retina into the sclerotomy is usually caused by excessively elevated intraocular pressure at the time of drainage. As already mentioned it is is one of the causes of a dry tap although occasionally, after an initial appearance of SRF, the flow will suddenly cease despite the fact that a large amount of SRF still remains in the eye. Ophthalmoscopy reveals a star-shaped puckering at the drainage site.

Prevention
1. Do not drain SRF when intraocular pressure is high by taking the following precautions:
   (a) Ensure the assistant is not pulling on the traction sutures.
   (b) Ensure the sutures are not tightened over the explant.
   (c) Ensure the encircling strap has not been tightened.
2. Drain over immobile retina (if possible).
3. Make a small perforation in the choroid which will allow a slow and gradual drainage of SRF.

Management
1. Apply pressure over the sclerotomy site with the tip of a squint hook in an attempt to reposit the incarcerated retina.
2. If incarceration is in the bed of the buckle, no further action is required if it cannot be reposited with the squint hook.
3. If incarceration is away from the bed of the buckle, support the incarcerated area of retina on a local buckle to prevent postoperative traction and possible persistence of SRF.

Vitreous prolapse

Causes
1. Attempted drainage at the site of flat retina: therefore always check the position of SRF immediately prior to drainage.
2. Drainage near a large break in which retrohyaloid fluid followed by solid vitreous passes through the break and

leaks out through the sclerotomy. This fairly rare complication may not always be preventable because it is not always possible to avoid drainage near a large break.

Management
1. Inspect the sclerotomy to make sure that there is no associated retinal incarceration – if incarceration is present, try to reposit the retina with the tip of a squint hook.
2. Excise the vitreous prolapse with scissors.
3. If the prolapse is in an area of flat retina, apply cryotherapy to the associated iatrogenic retinal tear.
4. If the prolapse is in an area of detached retina, take no further action.

Miscellaneous

1. **Damage to long posterior ciliary arteries and nerves** can be avoided by not draining SRF immediately under the horizontal recti; it is safe to drain just above or below.
2. **Postoperative bacterial endophthalmitis** – (see Chapter 9).

Intravitreal injections

Air injection

Indications

1. Severe ocular hypotony after drainage of SRF.
2. 'Fishmouthing' of a U-shaped tear (see Figure 8.27*a*).
3. Radial retinal folds.

Technique

1. Take a 25-gauge needle on a 5 ml syringe and make sure that both are dry to prevent the formation of small bubbles during injection.
2. Fill the syringe with air through a micropore filter.
3. With the toothed forceps grasp a muscle tendon and position the globe so that the injection site is uppermost.
4. Steady the globe and insert the needle 4 mm behind the limbus to avoid the vitreous base. Take care not to damage the long posterior ciliary arteries and nerves which run in the suprachoroidal space in line with the horizontal recti. If the eye is very soft following drainage of a large volume of SRF, a preliminary half-thickness scratch incision will facilitate the introduction of the needle without excessively deforming the globe.
5. While viewing through the pupil using the indirect ophthalmoscope without a condensing lens, aim the needle at the centre of the vitreous cavity and push it through the pars plana.

113

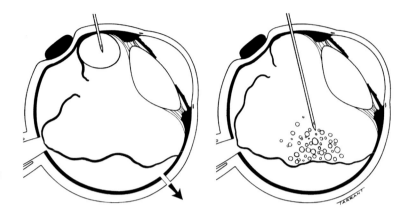

Figure 8.30 Injection of air into the vitreous cavity. *Left:* correct technique; *right:* incorrect technique

6. Do not pass the needle into the centre of the vitreous cavity but stop when the tip of the needle is just visible through the pupil. Make sure you have penetrated the non-pigmented epithelium of the pars plana.
7. Make a single smooth injection (Figure 8.30, left) and at the same time ask the assistant to check the intraocular pressure by depressing the cornea with a squint hook. The intraocular pressure should not exceed 30 mmHg; if necessary, check it with a Schiotz tonometer.
8. Quickly withdraw the needle; the incision is self-closing.
9. If the injection has been used to tamponade a large retinal tear, the patient should be appropriately positioned post-operatively.

Potential problems

Loss of fundus visualization
Loss of visualization of the fundus as a result of the formation of small air bubbles in the vitreous is the main disadvantage of air as compared with saline injection. This problem can be avoided by taking the following precautions:

1. Ensure that the syringe and needle are dry.
2. Inject with one movement of the plunger.
3. Do not introduce the needle into the centre of the vitreous cavity (Figure 8.30, *right*).
4. The injection site should be uppermost so that the initial few small bubbles collect and remain around the tip of the needle before coalescing into a single large bubble. The small bubbles will usually coalesce after a few minutes. They can also be made to move out of the way by repositioning the globe.

Excessive elevation of intraocular pressure
Excessive elevation of intraocular pressure by air injection is undesirable because it may result in corneal oedema, loss of

buckle height and anterior displacement of an iris-supported lens with damage to the corneal endothelium. It is therefore better to have an eye that is slightly too soft than too hard. Management is as follows:

1. Drain more SRF (if present), but there is a danger of retinal incarceration.
2. Aspirate air from the vitreous; this may be difficult if the cornea is oedematous.
3. Perform an anterior chamber paracentesis.

Miscellaneous
1. **Lens damage** can be avoided by taking into account the tilt of the globe and aiming the needle at the centre of the vitreous cavity and away from the lens.
3. **Retinal damage** may occur if the needle is inserted too posteriorly. Remember that the ora serrata is located 6 mm behind the limbus nasally and 7 mm temporally.
4. **Haemorrhage** is a rare complication resulting from damage to the long posterior ciliary arteries.
5. **Postoperative bacterial endophthalmitis** (see Chapter 9).

Saline injection

Indications
1. Severe ocular hypotony following drainage of SRF.
2. Radial retinal folds unassociated with 'fishmouthing'. Saline must not be used to tamponade a retinal tear because it will pass through the tear into the subretinal space.

Technique

The technique is the same as for air injection except that the needle should be introduced into the centre of the vitreous cavity before the injection is commenced.

Potential problems

These are the same as for air injection except:

1. Saline will not result in loss of visualization as air bubbles are not introduced into the eye.
2. Saline may pass through a retinal break and increase the amount of retinal elevation.

Pneumatic retinopexy

Pneumatic retinopexy is an out-patient procedure in which an intravitreal expanding gas bubble is used to seal a retinal break and reattach the retina without scleral buckling. The most

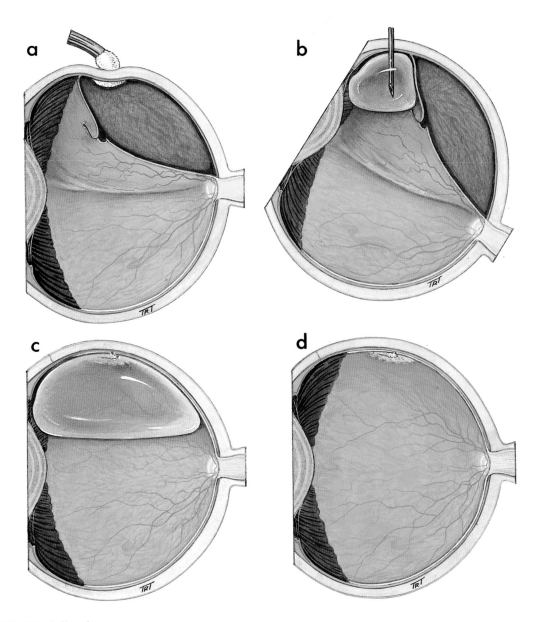

Figure 8.31 Principles of pneumatic retinopexy (see text)

frequently used gases are sulphur hexafluoride (SF6) and perfluoropropane (C3F8). The procedure is limited to treatment of uncomplicated RDs with a small retinal break or a cluster of breaks extending over an area of less than two clock hours situated in the upper two-thirds of the peripheral retina. The following two methods can be used depending on the amount of SRF.

Shallow SRF associated with a break which can be easily closed by scleral indentation

1. Prepare the eye with topical antibiotics, anaesthetic and 5% povidone-iodine.
2. Insert a speculum.
3. Treat the retinal breaks with cryotherapy (Figure 8.31a). Plenty of scleral indentation is helpful in reducing the intraocular pressure and thus facilitating the subsequent intravitreal injection of the gas bubble.
4. Inject into the vitreous cavity either 0.5 ml of 100% SF6 or 0.3 ml of 100% C3F8 (Figure 8.31b).
5. With forceps or a sterile cotton wool bud seal the scleral entry site to prevent the escape of gas under the conjunctiva.
6. Postoperatively position the patient's head so that the break is uppermost and the rising gas bubble in contact with the tear for 5-7 days (Figure 8.31c and d).

Moderately bullous RD associated with a break that cannot be closed by scleral indentation

1 and 2 As above.
3. Omit cryotherapy.
4–6 As above.
7. As soon as the retina flattens treat the breaks by laser photocoagulation, preferably using the indirect ophthalmoscopic delivery system because it is easier to apply through a gas bubble than slitlamp delivery.
8. Continue postoperative positioning for 5-7 days until adequate chorioretinal adhesion is established.

Completion of surgery

1. With two Moorfields forceps, identify the entire extent of the cut edge of the conjunctiva and Tenon's by starting at one end and working your way round (Figure 8.32).
2. Pull the edge of the conjunctiva and Tenon's to its original position at the limbus.
3. Close the radial relaxing incisions with one or two interrupted 6/0 plain catgut or polyglactin 9/0 (Vicryl) sutures. Bury the knots by beginning the suture on the scleral side of Tenon's. The cut ends of the conjunctiva and Tenon's should be about 2 mm posterior to the limbus (Figure 8.33) because by the first postoperative day they will have moved anteriorly to the limbus. If they are sutured to lie at the limbus, they will still move anteriorly onto the cornea and may interfere with postoperative ophthalmoscopy.
4. Trim redundant conjunctiva and Tenon's with scissors.
5. Inject 20 mg of gentamicin and 2 mg of betamethasone under Tenon's capsule, preferably in the same quadrant as the explant.
6. Pad the eye to lessen postoperative chemosis.

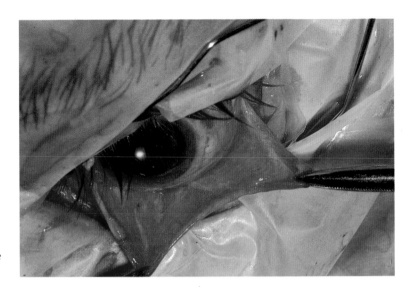

Figure 8.32 Identification of the cut edges of the conjunctiva and Tenon's capsule

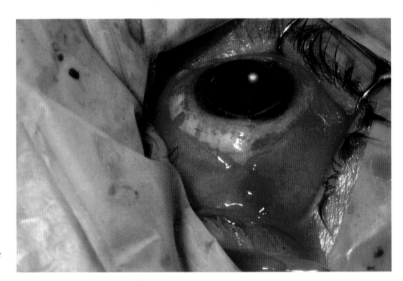

Figure 8.33 Final position of the conjunctiva

7. Examine the fellow eye carefully with scleral indentation and, if necessary, prophylactically treat with cryotherapy or indirect ophthalmoscopic laser photocoagulation any predisposing lesions.

Postoperative notes

For future reference it is important to have an adequate record of the operative procedure. This can usually be documented by a schematic sketch. The following points should be noted:

118

1. Extent and type of scleral buckling.
2. Site of drainage of SRF is marked with an 'X'.
3. Site of the Watzke sleeve.
4. Site of the intravitreal injection.
5. Intraoperative complications such as choroidal haemorrhage, retinal incarceration, vitreous prolapse etc.
6. State of the retina at the end of the procedure; flat or still some SRF remaining.
7. Antibiotic injections; mainly for medicolegal reasons.
8. Clinical features of the fellow eye and details of any prophylactic treatment. It is important to record negative findings such as the fellow eye having been examined with scleral indentation but no predisposing lesions detected.

Clinical examples

The following clinical examples will emphasize the most important aspects of management just discussed.

Fresh retinal detachment

Preoperative considerations

Examination shows a localized right upper temporal RD due to a U-tear (Figure 8.34*a*). The prognosis for central vision is good because the macula is uninvolved. The patient should be admitted immediately, rested flat in bed and operated on as soon as possible because the macula is in great danger for two reasons:
(a) The break is located in the upper temporal quadrant.
(b) SRF will spread quickly because the break is large.

Surgical technique

1. **Peritomy** should extend from 8.30 to 12.30 o'clock to expose the lateral and superior recti.
2. **Buckling**: most U-tears can be sealed with a 5 mm sponge explant (Figure 8.34*b*). The sutures should be about 8 mm apart to obtain adequate height to the buckle. The buckle should be placed radially to prevent the possibility of 'fishmouthing'. Figure 8.34*c* shows an undersized buckle. Accurate positioning of the explant is vital in this case. Figure 8.34*d* shows a malpositioned buckle.
3. **Drainage of SRF** may not be required because:
   (a) The retina is freely mobile.
   (b) The break can be apposed to RPE without difficulty.
   (c) The SRF is watery because the RD is fresh.
   It should be remembered that great care should be taken not to occlude the central retinal artery during a non-drainage procedure.

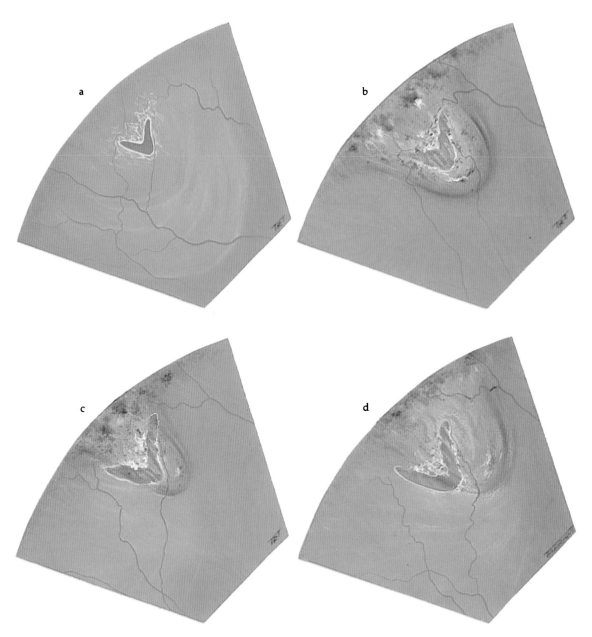

Figure 8.34 Management of a fresh upper temporal retinal detachment (see text)

Long-standing retinal detachment

Preoperative considerations

Examination shows an extensive right RD with macular involvement associated with a U-tear in the upper temporal quadrant and two small round holes in the lower temporal quadrant (Figure 8.35*a*). A partially pigmented demarcation line

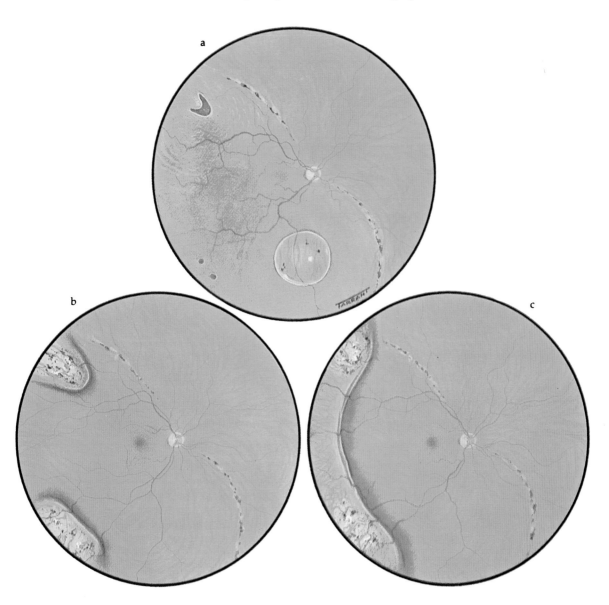

Figure 8.35 Management of a
long-standing retinal
detachment (see text)

is present at the junction of detached and flat retina, and a
secondary intraretinal cyst is present inferiorly. This is therefore
a long-standing RD because demarcation marks take about 3
months to develop and secondary retinal cysts usually take
about 12 months. The prognosis for restoration of good visual
acuity is very poor because the fovea has probably been
detached for at least 12 months. There is therefore no urgency
for surgery, which can be performed at the patient's and
surgeon's convenience.

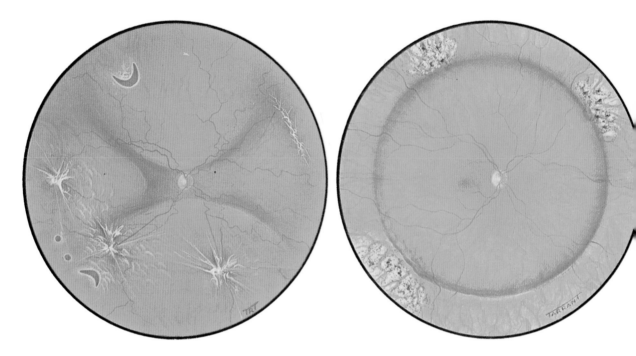

Figure 8.36 Mangement of a total retinal detachment associated with proliferative vitreoretinopathy (see text)

Surgical technique

1. **Peritomy** should extend from 5.30 to 12.30 o'clock to expose the superior, lateral and inferior recti.
2. **Buckling**: the U-tear can be sealed with a 5 mm-wide radial explant and the two holes with a 4 mm-wide circumferential explant (Figure 8.35*b*). Alternatively, all breaks can be sealed with a long 4 mm-wide circumferential sponge explant extending from 7 to 10.30 o'clock (Figure 8.35*c*).
3. **Drainage of SRF** is probably required because in long-standing cases SRF is viscous and may take a long time to absorb.

Retinal detachment associated with moderate PVR

Preoperative considerations

Examination shows a total right RD, with breaks and lattice degeneration in three separate quadrants (Figure 8.36, *left*). Star-shaped retinal folds present in two quadrants of detached retina are indicative of moderate PVR. The prognosis for restoration of good visual acuity is not good because the macula is involved and the presence of PVR reduces the prognosis for reattachment.

Surgical technique

1. **Peritomy** should extend for 360° to expose all four recti.
2. **Buckling** should involve an encircling procedure because retinal breaks and lattice degeneration involve three quadrants of the detached retina. A permanent buckle is also desirable because PVR is present. The buckling material can be either a 3 or 4 mm sponge (Figure 8.36, *right*) or a strap supplemented by a hard silicone tyre to support the retinal breaks.
3. **Drainage of SRF** is necessary to close the breaks because the retina is not freely mobile.

Further reading

Brown, P. and Chignell, A. H. (1982) Accidental drainage of subretinal fluid. *British Journal of Ophthalmology*, **66**, 625–626

Chen, J. C., Robertson, J. E., Coonan, P. *et al.* (1988) Results and complications of pneumatic retinopexy. *Ophthalmology*, **95**, 601–608

Chignell, A. H. (1977) Retinal mobility in retinal detachment surgery. *British Journal of Ophthalmology*, **61**, 446–449

Chignell, A. H. and Markham, R. H. G. (1978) Buckling procedures and drainage of subretinal fluid. *Transactions of the Ophthalmological Society of the UK*, **97**, 474–477

Gilbert, C. and McLeod, D. (1985) D-ACE surgical sequence for selected bullous retinal detachments. *British Journal of Ophthalmology*, **69**, 729–732

Hilton, G. F. and Grizzard, W. S. (1986) Pneumatic retinopexy: a two step outpatient operation without a conjunctival incision. *Ophthalmology*, **93**, 626–641

Michels, R.G. (1986) Scleral buckling methods in rhegmatogenous retinal detachment. *Retina*, **6**, 1–49

Smiddy, W. E., Glaser, B. M., Michels, R. G. *et al.* (1990) Scleral buckle revision to treat rhegmatogenous retinal detachment. *Ophthalmic Surgery*, **21**, 716–720

Thompson, J. T. (1990) The repair of rhegmatogenous retinal detachment. *Ophthalmology*, **97**, 1562–1572

Tornambe, P. E. (1988) Pneumatic retinopexy. *Survey of Ophthalmology*, **32**, 270–281

Wilkinson, C. P. and Bradford, R. H. (1984) Complications of drainage of subretinal fluid. *Retina*, **4**, 1–4

Worsely, D. R. and Grey, R. H. B. (1991) Supplemental gas tamponade after conventional scleral buckling surgery: a simple alternative to surgical revision. *British Journal of Ophthalmology*, **75**, 535–537

9 Postoperative considerations

125

Early considerations

Routine management

The pad is removed on the first day and, unless the lids are excessively oedematous, the fundus is examined. A +30D lens is particularly useful in obtaining a general overall view. A slitlamp examination is then performed and the intraocular pressure measured. It is common to find a degree of lid oedema (Figure 9.1), conjunctival hyperaemia, moderate chemosis, dellen formation, mild filamentary keratopathy and mild anterior uveitis.

In the absence of complications most patients can be discharged on the first postoperative day and given a follow-up appointment for about 10-14 days. In the meantime they should use 1% atropine drops twice daily and a combination of a steroid and antibiotic drop (e.g. Betnesol-N or Maxitrol) for 3-4 weeks. After discharge they can resume normal activities but, although not strictly essential, most patients are happy to take 2 weeks off work. As mentioned in the previous chapter, certain patients with intravitreal air or gas may be required to posture face-down continuously for 5-7 days until an adequate chorioretinal adhesion has formed.

Absorption of subretinal fluid

Following drainage of SRF, the retina should be flat or very nearly flat on the first postoperative day and should remain flat thereafter. Following a non-drainage procedure, the volume of SRF should decrease each day so that the retina is flat by the third or fourth day.

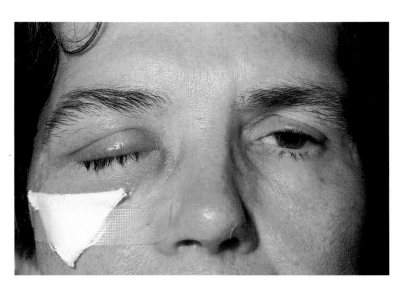

Figure 9.1 Oedema of eyelids on the first day following retinal detachment surgery

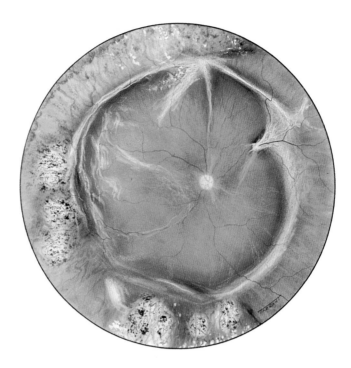

Figure 9.2 Postoperative persistence of a shallow retinal detachment due to severe vitreoretinal traction

Reaccumulation of SRF

Reaccumulation of SRF following drainage or an increase in volume after non-drainage is caused by one of the following:

1. **An open break** which has not been sealed at the time of surgery is by far the most common cause.
2. **Exudative RD** resulting from excessive cryotherapy is rare. It is important not to re-operate in these cases because the SRF will absorb spontaneously within 1 or 2 weeks.

Slow absorption of SRF

In some cases the SRF does not increase in volume but either fails to diminish or absorbs very slowly despite the fact that all breaks are closed. This may be caused by one of the following:

1. **Viscous SRF** in eyes with long-standing RD that have not been drained.
2. **Deficient RPE** in eyes with a hypopigmented fundus may be responsible for slow absorption of SRF. The collection of SRF is invariably located inferiorly and eventually absorbs after several weeks. In the meantime the patient should be advised to sleep with the head elevated in order to prevent spread of SRF to the fovea.
3. **Residual tractional RD** in eyes with fixed folds or severe vitreoretinal traction (Figure 9.2). In these cases a localized

127

fold of elevated retina may persist postoperatively for a variable period of time.

Causes of early failure

By far the most common cause of failure to reattach the retina is an open retinal break. The causes can be preoperative or operative.

Preoperative causes

It should be emphasized that about 50% of all RDs are associated with more than one break. In most cases the breaks are located within 90° of each other. At surgery, the surgeon should therefore not be satisfied if only one break has been found until a thorough search has been made for the presence of other breaks and the configuration of the RD corresponds to the position of the primary break (see Figure 2.21). In eyes with hazy media or intraocular lens implants, visualization of the peripheral retina may be difficult and all retinal breaks impossible to detect. As a last resort, the possibility of a hole at or near the posterior pole such as a true macular hole should be considered if no peripheral breaks can be detected.

Operative causes

The main operative causes of failure to seal all breaks are as follows:

1. **Buckle failure** may be the result of the following:
    (a) Buckle of inadequate size (see Figure 8.34*c*) – replace.
    (b) Buckle incorrectly positioned (see Figure 8.34*d*) – reposition.
    (c) Buckle of inadequate height – drain SRF if necessary.
2. **'Fishmouthing'** of the retinal tear which may or may not be associated with a communicating radial retinal fold (see Figure 8.27*a*). In some cases the tear can be closed by applying photocoagulation to the retina around the tear in order to induce swelling. If this is not successful, pneumatic retinopexy should be tried. Alternatively, reoperation may be necessary to reposition the explant (see Figure 8.27*b*).
3. **A missed iatrogenic break** caused inadvertently during drainage of SRF. Unless the new break is detected and treated at the time of initial surgery it must be sealed subsequently.

Complications

Acute orbital cellulitis

This rare complication is the result of insertion of contaminated buckling material. To prevent this complication some surgeons soak the buckling material in a bath containing an antibiotic.

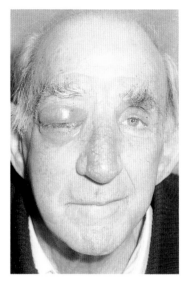

Figure 9.3 Orbital cellulitis following retinal detachment surgery

Clinical features

Presentation is during the first few days with pain and proptosis.

Examination shows the following: the eyelids are swollen, erythematous and warm and tender to palpation (Figure 9.3). Attempted ocular movements are painful. In advanced cases visual acuity may be diminished and there may be an increasing afferent pupillary conduction defect. The patient is unwell and pyrexial.

Differential diagnosis includes: (a) an abnormal reaction to surgery following extensive and prolonged procedures and (b) bacterial endophthalmitis.

Anterior segment ischaemia

This rare complication is caused by impairment of blood supply to the anterior segment by one of the following two causes:

1. **Excessive constriction of the globe** by a narrow and relatively posterior encircling band (Figure 9.4) which may impair the arterial blood supply via the long posterior ciliary arteries and also impede venous drainage via the vortex veins. Patients with SC sickle haemoglobinopathy are at particular risk.
2. **Disinsertion of two or more muscles** which may interfere with anterior segment blood supply via the anterior ciliary arteries, which are the terminal branches of the muscular

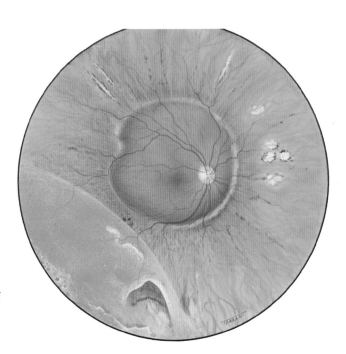

Figure 9.4 Very posterior encirclement with persistence of retinal detachment anterior to the buckle associated with a large open U-tear at 6 o'clock

arteries to the rectus muscles. Because muscle disinsertion is seldom necessary this is a rare cause.

Clinical features

Presentation is between the second and fifth day with mild to moderate pain.

Examination of mild cases shows chemosis, a usually low intraocular pressure and striate keratopathy with a few keratic precipitates. In severe cases there is stromal thickening and epithelial oedema. Flare and cells are universal; in severe cases, large pieces of fibrin float in the aqueous, and occasionally a hyphaema may develop as a result of venous congestion. There may also be pigment on the anterior lens capsule and anterior subcapsular opacities similar to 'glaukomflecken' seen in acute congestive glaucoma.

Differential diagnosis includes: (a) secondary angle-closure glaucoma – but the intraocular pressure is not raised and the anterior chamber is usually abnormally deep and (b) bacterial endophthalmitis.

Treatment

Treatment is empirical and frequently unsatisfactory. Mild cases may resolve with the help of topical steroids (dexamethasone drops hourly). Severe cases should be treated with both topical and systemic steroids and removal of the encircling band. Intravenous administration of a low molecular weight dextran (dextran 40, Rheomacrodex) may be beneficial if given early over a 24-hour period. In most cases, however, the prognosis is poor and many eyes subsequently develop corneal neovascularization, iris atrophy and occasionally rubeosis, and mature cataract.

Vitritis

Vitritis is caused by excessive cryotherapy due to one of the following mistakes:

1. **Failure to detect the end-point correctly** in eyes with bullous RDs, resulting in excessively long applications.
2. **Treatment or accidental re-treatment** of large areas of the retina.

Clinical features

Presentation is usually after the fourth day (later than infection) with slight pain, hazy vision and increase in small floaters.

Examination initially shows a vitreous haze which is most intense adjacent to the area of the buckle. Subsequently it spreads throughout the vitreous cavity. Early retinal findings consist of oedema at the sites of excessive freezing and occasionally a self-limiting exudative RD. Subsequently there is severe atrophy of the overtreated RPE and choroid (Figure 9.5). The

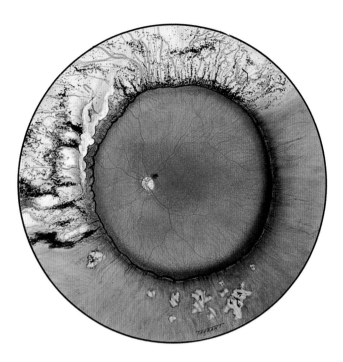

Figure 9.5 Very severe chorioretinal atrophy caused by excessive cryotherapy

dispersion of pigment derived from the RPE into the subretinal space at the time of cryotherapy may result in the subsequent development of multiple subretinal polymorphic black spots. The pigment may also cause a pseudodemarcation line along the border between previously detached and flat retina.

Differential diagnosis includes early bacterial endophthalmitis.

Treatment

Topical and posterior sub-Tenon's injection of betamethasone are usually effective in reducing the severity of vitritis. In very severe cases the use of systemic steroids should be considered.

Choroidal detachment

Choroidal detachment is a fairly common and usually innocuous complication caused by transudation of choroidal fluid into the potential space between the sclera and uvea (suprachoroidal space). The two main predisposing factors are the following:

1. **Prolonged severe ocular hypotony** which is invariably associated with drainage of a large volume of SRF. This causes a temporary insufficiency of the choroidal vasculature, resulting in transudation.
2. **Damage to vortex veins**, particularly by large posteriorly placed buckles, may occasionally be a contributory factor.

131

Postoperative considerations

Clinical features

Presentation is during the first three days but symptoms are usually absent.

Examination shows choroidal detachments (see Figure 4.15). The intraocular pressure is usually low although in some cases it may be high as a result of secondary angle closure.

Treatment

Most cases resolve spontaneously within 2 weeks and do not require treatment. There is no evidence that steroids (topical or systemic) or mydriatics have any beneficial effects in speeding up resolution. Surgical intervention is indicated in the very rare event of intractable secondary angle-closure glaucoma. The technique is as follows:

1. Drain suprachoroidal fluid through a small pars plana incision.
2. Reconstitute the intraocular volume by injecting saline into the vitreous cavity. If a retinal break is open, air injection is preferred.

Elevation of intraocular pressure

Severe elevation of intraocular pressure is rare. A secondary angle-closure glaucoma may occur as a result of shallowing of the anterior chamber caused by forward displacement of the iris-lens diaphragm and anterior rotation of the ciliary body. This is particularly likely to occur in eyes with pre-existing shallow anterior chambers in which a tight encircling procedure (see Figure 9.4) has obstructed the vortex veins.

Clinical features

Presentation is usually on the first day with pain and impaired vision.

Examination shows raised intraocular pressure, a shallow anterior chamber and variable epithelial oedema.

Differential diagnosis includes primary angle-closure glaucoma induced by mydriatics.

Treatment

The intraocular pressure should be reduced with oral carbonic anhydrase inhibitors and topical aqueous suppressants. In severe cases, oral glycerol or intravenous mannitol, may be required but pilocarpine and laser iridotomy are ineffective. Topical treatment is with atropine to induce cycloplegia and mydriasis, and steroids to prevent formation of posterior synechiae. With this conservative treatment the intraocular pressure is usually controlled and cutting of the encircling strap is seldom required.

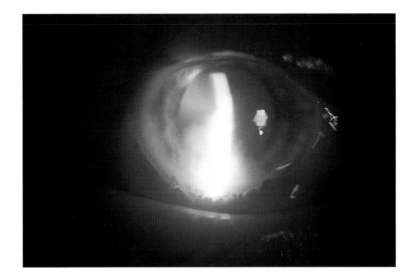

Figure 9.6 Postoperative bacterial endophthalmitis

Bacterial endophthalmitis

Bacterial endophthalmitis is fortunately very uncommon following retinal surgery. Predisposing factors include the following:

1. Entry of bacteria through the drainage site.
2. Introduction of bacteria into the eye during intravitreal injection.
3. Rarely, entry of bacteria through necrotic sclera.

Presentation is usually within 24-48 hours with pain and severe progressive loss of vision.
Examination of severe cases shows lid oedema, chemosis, corneal haze, fibrinous exudate or hypopyon in the anterior chamber (Figure 9.6), vitritis, an absent red reflex and inability to visualize the fundus with the indirect ophthalmoscope. However, in mild or early cases some of the above features may be absent. Details of management are beyond the scope of this book.

Late considerations

Routine management

Both eyes should be examined with the slitlamp and indirect ophthalmoscope at each visit. Topical therapy can usually be discontinued 4 weeks postoperatively. The next outpatient visit is for 3 months, when any change in refraction induced by the operation should have stabilized and a new prescription ordered. The patient is seen again 6 months later and then annually. The patient should be encouraged to return immedi-

133

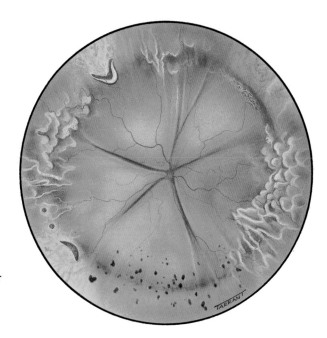

Figure 9.7 Total retinal detachment associated with proliferative vitreoretinopathy following an initially successful encirclement – note open U-tear at 11 o'clock with rolled edges and pigment clumps on the inferior retina

ately he notices any new symptom such as photopsia, floaters or diminished vision. However, persistent photopsia may persist for months and even years in patients with perfectly flat retinae.

Causes of late failure

Late failure is defined as initial reattachment of the retina and subsequent re-detachment after discharge.

Proliferative vitreoretinopathy

The postoperative development of PVR is the most common cause of late failure. The incidence of PVR is 8% after the first operation, 12% after the second and 18% after the third. The traction forces associated with PVR can open old breaks and create new ones.

Presentation is typically between the fourth and sixth postoperative weeks. After an initial period of visual improvement following successful retinal reattachment the patient reports a sudden and progressive loss of vision, which may develop within a few hours.

Examination usually shows severe (Grade C) PVR (Figure 9.7).

Reopening of retinal break

A retinal break may reopen in the absence of PVR as a result of either (a) **inadequate technique** or (b) **late buckle failure**.

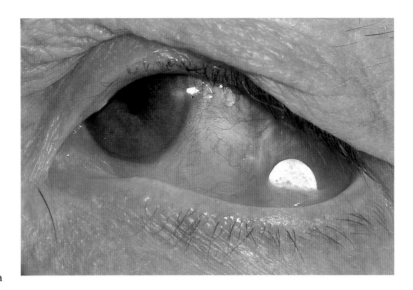

Figure 9.8 Erosion of sponge explant through the conjunctiva

Inadequate technique

1. **Inadequate cryotherapy**: small round holes do not usually leak postoperatively, even if they have not been adequately treated by cryotherapy, provided they are located on the buckle. U-tears of moderate to large dimensions may leak postoperatively even though they are initially closed by the buckle, unless they are well surrounded by cryotherapy. This is because persistent traction on the flap of the tear may pull the sensory retina away from the RPE and allow SRF to reaccumulate.
2. **Inadequate buckling** of the vitreous base anterior to the retinal tear may result in reopening of the tear and anterior leakage of SRF.

Late buckle failure

The following are the main causes of late buckle failure.

1. **Slipping** of an encircling element anteriorly or posteriorly.
2. **Loosening** of the encircling element.
3. **Spontaneous extrusion** of the explant.
4. **Removal** of the explant because of infection or exposure.

New break formation

Occasionally, new retinal breaks develop in areas of the retina subjected to persistent vitreoretinal traction following local buckling. This is less likely to occur following encircling procedures which give a permanent buckle. New inferior retinal breaks can form as a result of upward vitreous traction induced by an expanding intravitreal gas bubble following pneumatic retinopexy.

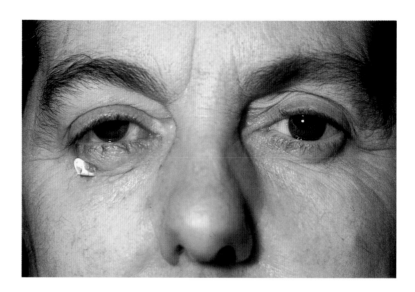

Figure 9.9 Erosion of sponge explant through the lower eyelid

Complications

Exposure of explant

The explant, usually a sponge, may become exposed several weeks or months postoperatively. It usually cuts through the conjunctiva and Tenon's (Figure 9.8) although very rarely it may erode through one of the eyelids (Figure 9.9). The following are the main causes:

1. Inadequate coverage of the explant with Tenon's capsule and conjunctiva during closure.
2. Inadequate suturing of the explant to the sclera.
3. Failure to trim the ends of the explant so a sharp edge erodes through the conjunctiva.
4. Large sponge placed too anteriorly.

Clinical features

Presentation is after a variable time following surgery. The patient reports a chronic discharge and seeing something white in the eye. Some patients may report that the explant has dropped out altogether.
Examination shows an exposed explant which may be associated with chronic conjunctivitis.

Treatment

1. Spontaneous complete extrusion of an explant requires no specific treatment apart from the administration of a short course of topical antibiotics until the conjunctiva has healed.

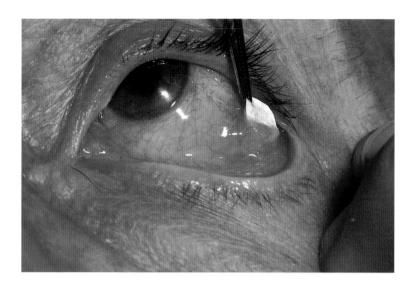

Figure 9.10 Sponge explant grasped with forceps

2. A partially extruded small and loosely attached explant can simply be pulled out with forceps (Figures 9.10, 9.11) after the instillation of topical anaesthetic.
3. Large partially extruded sponges which are still tightly attached to the sclera may require a general anaesthetic for removal.

Removal of a buckle during the first few months postoperatively is associated with a 5–10% risk of re-detachment.

Infection of explant

Although rare, late infection is more common than acute early infection.
Presentation is with pain and tenderness.
Examination shows erythema over the explant, subconjunctival haemorrhages, local granuloma, chronic conjunctivitis or a fistula.
Treatment requires removal of the contaminated material.

Migration of encircling strap

Very occasionally an encircling strap may migrate anteriorly and even cut through the tendons of the rectus muscles. Migration into the globe may also rarely occur.

Clinical features

Presentation of internal migration of an encircling element is usually with recurrent vitreous haemorrhage as a result of damage to the sensory retina. Retinal re-detachment may occur in advanced cases.

137

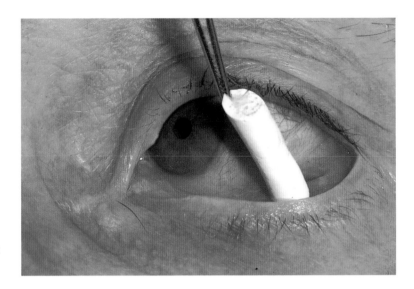

Figure 9.11 Removal of sponge explant

Examination of the fundus shows a shining appearance of the encircling element.

Treatment

Treatment is difficult because it is important not to inflict more complications by trying to remove the encircling element than by leaving it alone. The main indication for removal is recurrent and severe vitreous haemorrhage and/or recurrence of RD. The technique is as follows:

1. Identify the sites of entry and exit of the band.
2. Cut the band at one site and carefully remove it by sliding it out. Make sure that any discontinuities such as sutures do not erode the retina. It may be sufficient merely to cut the band and leave it *in situ*.

Maculopathy

Following successful surgery the macula may appear clinically normal or the following specific changes may be seen which may or may not be associated with impaired visual acuity.

1. **Cellophane maculopathy** is characterized by an abnormal reflex at the macula which is not associated with distortion of the surrounding blood vessels. This finding is compatible with normal visual acuity.
2. **Macular pucker** is characterized by an opaque membrane and distortion of blood vessels (see Figure 5.3). It is a more advanced stage of cellophane maculopathy caused by the proliferation and subsequent contraction of an epiretinal membrane. This complication appears to be related neither

to the type, extent or duration of RD, nor to the type of surgical procedure, and it may rarely occur following prophylactic treatment. Most eyes with macular pucker have a visual acuity of less than 6/18.

3. **Pigmentary maculopathy** is usually caused by pigment fallout as a result of excessive cryotherapy. Visual acuity, however, is usually unimpaired.

4. **Cystoid macular oedema** is much less common than following cataract extraction but it has a more prolonged course. In persistent cases, visual acuity is usually less than 6/12.

5. **Cystoid macular degeneration** unassociated with leakage of fluorescein from the perifoveal capillaries typically occurs in eyes with long-standing involvement of the macula by SRF. Visual acuity is usually very poor, and when the cystoid changes resolve they are replaced by degenerative lesions involving the RPE without any improvement in visual function.

6. **Macular hole** is seen occasionally and is associated with a visual acuity of less than 6/36.

7. **Atrophic maculopathy** is usually caused by the gravitation of blood in the subretinal space due to intraoperative choroidal haemorrhage.

8. **Delayed absorption of SRF at the macula** which may persist for many months and simulate a detachment of the RPE.

Extraocular muscle imbalance

Transient diplopia is fairly common during the immediate postoperative period and is a good prognostic sign indicating macular re-attachment. Persistent diplopia is rare and may require strabismus surgery or botulinum toxin injection. The following are the main predisposing factors for diplopia:

1. **A large sponge** inserted under one of the rectus muscles. In most cases the diplopia resolves spontaneously after a few weeks or months and requires no specific therapy apart from reassurance or the temporary use of prisms. Very rarely the sponge has to be removed.

2. **Surgical disinsertion** of a rectus muscle (usually superior or inferior rectus) in order to place a buckle under the muscle. This is now a rare cause of diplopia as muscle disinsertion is usually unnecessary.

3. **Rupture of the muscle belly** as a result of excessive traction on the sutures. This may cause a complete and severe palsy unless the cut ends can be approximated. Treatment may be very difficult and requires muscle operations on both eyes.

4. **Severe conjunctival scarring**, usually associated with repeated operations, may cause mechanical restriction of eye movements.

5. **Decompensation of a large heterophoria** resulting from poor postoperative visual acuity in the operated eye.

Miscellaneous

1. **Changes in refraction**: local buckles may induce mild astigmatism while encircling buckles may induce myopia which averages 2.75D by increasing the axial length of the globe. The induced changes in refraction are usually stable by about the fourth month.
2. **Ptosis** may occur, particularly in elderly patients, due to postoperative stretching of an already attenuated levator aponeurosis by lid oedema. The ptosis is usually mild and can be corrected with a Fasanella-Servat procedure.
3. **Cataract**, which is uncommon, may be caused by one of the following:
    (a) Lens injury during intravitreal injections.
    (b) Anterior segment necrosis.
    (c) Progression of pre-existing lens opacities.
    (d) Persistent RD.

Further reading

Chignell, A. H., Revie, I. H. S. and Clemett, R. S. (1971) Complications of retinal cryotherapy. *Transactions of the Ophthalmological Society of the UK*, **91**, 635–651

Cleary, P. E. and Leaver, P. K. (1978) Macular abnormalities in the reattached retina. *British Journal of Ophthalmology*, **62**, 595–603

Fison, P. M. and Chignell, A. H. (1987) Diplopia after retinal detachment surgery. *British Journal of Ophthalmology*, **71**, 521–525

Goel, R., Crewdson, J. and Chignell, A. H. (1983) Astigmatism following retinal detachment surgery. *British Journal of Ophthalmology*, , **67**, 327–329

Hahan, Y. S., Lincoff, A., Lincoff, H. *et al.* (1979) Infection after sponge implantation for scleral buckling. *American Journal of Ophthalmology*, **87**, 180–185

Hilton, C. F. (1974) Subretinal pigment migration; effects of cryosurgical retinal reattachment. *Archives of Ophthalmology*, **91**, 445–450

Hilton, G. F. and Wallyn, R. H. (1979) The removal of scleral buckles. *Archives of Ophthalmology*, **96**, 2061–2063

Kanski, J. J., Elkington, A. R. and Davies, M. S. (1973) Diplopia after retinal detachment surgery. *American Journal of Ophthalmology*, **76**, 38–40

Sabates, N. R., Sabates, F. N., Sabates, R. *et al.* (1989) Macular changes after retinal detachment surgery. *American Journal of Ophthalmology*, , **108**, 22–29

Schwartz, P. L. and Pruett, R. C. (1977) Factors influencing retinal detachment after removal of buckling elements. *Archives of Ophthalmology*, **95**, 804–808

Smiddy, W. E., Loupe, D., Michels, R. G. *et al.* (1989) Extraocular muscle imbalance after scleral buckling surgery. *Archives of Ophthalmology*, **107**, 1469–1471

Wiznia, R. A. (1983) Removal of solid silicone rubber explants after retinal detachment surgery. *American Journal of Ophthalmology*, **95**, 495–497

Yoshizumi, M. O. (1980) Exposure of intrascleral implants. *Ophthalmology*, **87**, 1150–1154

10 Principles of vitrectomy for retinal detachment

Main aims of vitrectomy

Instrumentation

Tamponading agents
  Expanding gases
  Heavy liquids
  Silicone oils

Indications for vitrectomy
  Rhegmatogenous retinal detachments
  Tractional retinal detachments

Main aims of vitrectomy

Vitrectomy is a microsurgical procedure designed to remove vitreous gel, usually in order to gain access to a diseased retina. The most common approach is via three separate incisions in the pars plana. The following are the main aims of vitrectomy in the management of RD:

1. **Removal of vitreous opacities**, if present.
2. **Excision of the posterior hyaloid face** (PHF) up to the posterior border of the vitreous base is of paramount importance in eyes with RD. The so called 'core' vitrectomy which leaves the PHF and any associated retinal membranes intact is justifiable only in the managmenet of endophthalmitis.
3. **Relief of vitreoretinal traction** by epiretinal membrane dissection and/or retinotomy.
4. **Retinal manipulation and re-attachment**.
5. **Creation of a space** within the vitreous cavity for subsequent internal tamponade.
6. **Miscellaneous aims**, where appropriate, include removal of associated cataract, dislocated lens fragments or intraocular foreign bodies.

Instrumentation

The instrumentation is complex and, in addition to the vitreous cutter, many other instruments must be available. The diameter of the shafts of most instruments is 0.9 (20-gauge) so that they are interchangable and can be inserted through either sclerotomy.

1. **The cutter** has an inner guillotine blade which oscillates up to 800 times/minute (Figure 10.1). This minimizes any transvitreal traction on the retina during surgery. The vitreous gel is cut into small pieces and simultaneously removed by suction into a collecting bottle.

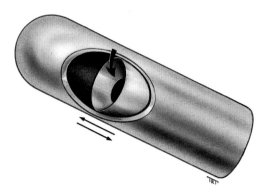

Figure 10.1 Vitreous cutter

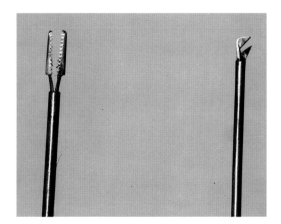

Figure 10.2 *Left:* forceps; *right:* vertically cutting scissors

2. **The intraocular illumination source** is through a 20-gauge fibreoptic probe which delivers light from an 80–150 watt bulb.
3. **The infusion cannula** usually has an intraocular length of 4 mm although in special circumstances such as aphakic or pseudophakic eyes with opaque media a 6 mm cannula may be required.
4. **Accessory instruments** include:
   (a) Vitreous scissors which can cut either vertically (Figure 10.2, *top*) for segmentation or horizontally for delamination of epiretinal membranes.
   (b) Vitreous forceps (Figure 10.2, *bottom*).
   (c) Backflush flute needle.
   (d) Endodiathermy, endolaser and laser delivery via an indirect ophthalmoscope.

Tamponading agents

The two main purposes of internal tamponage are:

1. To achieve hydraulic intraoperative retinal flattening by internal drainage of SRF and fluid-gas exchange.
2. To produce internal closure of retinal breaks during the postoperative period.

The ideal tamponading agent should have a high surface tension, be optically clear and biologically inert. In the absence of such ideal substance the following are in current use:

Expanding gases

Although air can be used in certain cases one of the following expanding gases is usually preferred in order to achieve prolonged intraocular tamponade:

143

1. **Sulphur hexafluoride** (SF6) which doubles its volume and lasts 10–14 days.
2. **Perfluoroethane** (C2F6) which triples its volume and lasts 30–35 days.
3. **Perfluoropropane** (C3F8) which quadruples its volume and lasts 55–65 days.

Heavy liquids

Heavy liquids (perfluorocarbons) have a high specific gravity and thus remain in a dependent position when injected into the vitreous cavity. The main indications are as follows:

1. To stabilize the posterior retina during epiretinal membrane dissection in eyes with PVR.
2. To unfold a giant retinal tear.
3. To remove posteriorly dislocated lens fragments or intraocular lens implants.

Silicone oils

Silicone oils have a low specific gravity and are thus buoyant. They allow for more controlled intraoperative retinal manipulation and may also be used for prolonged postoperative intraocular tamponade. The most commonly used liquid silicones have relatively low viscosity (1000–5000 cs). The 1000 cs silicone is easy to inject and to remove whilst 5000 cs silicone is less prone to the production of tiny droplets (emulsification). However, variation in viscosity is unrelated to surface tension.

Indications for vitrectomy

Although there are many indications for vitrectomy only those relating to retinal detachment surgery will be mentioned. Vitrectomy techniques can be used in the treatment of selected rhegmatogenous RDs and for most tractional RD.

Rhegmatogenous retinal detachments

It must be stressed that the vast majority of rhegmatogenous RD can be treated successfully by scleral buckling techniques as already described. Vitrectomy is reserved for the following two types of cases.

Inability to visualize the causative break

1. **Vitreous opacities** such as blood, debris and occasionally asteroid hyalosis. Dense vitreous haemorrhage is frequently associated with a large posterior retinal break.

2. **Internal search** for hidden retinal breaks.
3. **A thickened posterior capsule** in pseudophakic eyes (see Figure 6.4) that may require capsulectomy.

Inability to close breaks by standard techniques

A scleral buckling procedure should be performed only if there is high probability of a successful outcome. A 'trial of scleral buckling' or 'blind encirclement' should not be undertaken because it may result in persistent retinal detachment and acceleration of PVR which carries a much less favourable visual prognosis. The main indications for vitrectomy in this category are the following:

1. **Very large breaks** including giant tears (see Figure 3.11, *bottom*).
2. **Posterior breaks** including macular holes (see Figure 4.4).
3. **Severe vitreoretinal traction** as in proliferative vitreoretinopathy (see Figure 4.9).

The main advantages of primary vitrectomy in such cases are:

1. Reduction of ocular manipulation as a scleral buckle can be small or may not be required at all.
2. Retinopexy (cryotherapy or laser) is more controlled as it is applied after the retina has been re-attached intraoperatively and the amount of destructive energy is reduced to a minimum.
3. A tamponading agent ensures postoperative internal closure of the retinal break.

Tractional retinal detachments

The cause of RD in this category is contraction of epiretinal membranes (usually preretinal, only rarely subretinal) rather than retinal breaks. Scleral buckling procedures cannot effectively eliminate traction due to epiretinal membranes so that vitrectomy combined with epiretinal membrane dissection is the procedure of choice. The two main causes of tractional RD are: (a) **advanced proliferative diabetic retinopathy** and (b) **penetrating trauma of the posterior segment**. A less common indication for vitrectomy is advanced retinopathy of prematurity.

Indications in advanced proliferative diabetic retinopathy

1. **Tractional RD involving or threatening the macula** (Figure 10.3, *left*). If necessary, vitrectomy can be combined with internal panretinal photocoagulation (Figure 10.3, *right*). Extramacular tractional RD may be observed because, in many cases, it may remain stationary for a long time.
2. **Combined traction and rhegmatogenous RD** should be treated urgently, even if the macula is not involved, because

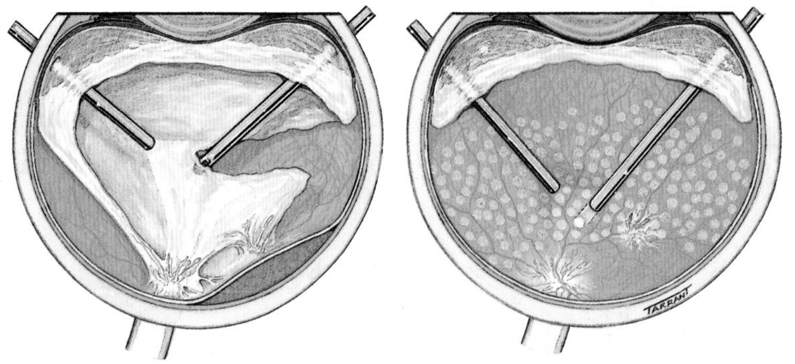

Figure 10.3 Principles of vitrectomy for tractional retinal detachment in severe proliferative diabetic retinopathy. *Left:* excision of traction on posterior retina; *right:* panretinal endophotocoagulation

SRF is likely to spread quickly to involve the macula.

It should be noted that, apart from RD, other indications for vitrectomy in advanced proliferative diabetic retinopathy include the following:

1. Recurrent and/or non-absorbing vitreous haemorrhage.
2. 'Early vitrectomy' when laser photocoagulation is either impossible or ineffective in controlling progression of fibrovascular proliferation.
3. Dense, persistent, premacular, subhyaloid haemorrhage.
4. Rubeosis associated with vitreous haemorrhage which is sufficiently dense to preclude panretinal photocoagulation.

Indications in penetrating trauma

1. **Prevention of tractional RD**: unlike diabetic retinopathy where epiretinal membrane proliferation occurs mostly on the posterior retina, fibrocellular proliferation after penetrating trauma tends to develop on the pre-equatorial retina and/or the ciliary body. Treatment is usually aimed at visual rehabilitation and minimizing the tractional process.
2. **Late tractional RD**, which is usually associated with an intraocular foreign body, may develop months after an otherwise successful removal of the foreign body.

Further reading

de Juan, E. Jr and Hickinbotham, D. (1990) Refinements in microinstrumentation for vitreous surgery. *American Journal of Ophthalmology* , **109**, 218–220

Fleischman, J., Lerner, B. C. and Reimels, H. (1989) A new intraocular aspiration probe with bipolar cautery and reflux capabilities. *Archives of Ophthalmology*, **107**, 283

Michels, R. G., Rice, T. A. and Ober, R. R. (1979) Vitreoretinal dissection instruments. *American Journal of Ophthalmology*

11 Vitrectomy techniques

Sclerotomies

Technique

1. Secure the infusion cannula to the sclera 3.5 mm behind the limbus at the level of the inferior border of a lateral rectus muscle.
2. Make two further sclerotomies at the 10 and 2 o'clock positions and temporarily close with plugs.

Potential problems

1. **Suprachoroidal or subretinal infusion** can be avoided by ensuring that the infusion port of the cannula has penetrated well into the vitreous cavity and is not covered by uveal tissue or retina. If the tip of the cannula has not cleanly entered the vitreous cavity the infusion fluid may enter the suprachoroidal or subretinal space. This is more likely to occur in hypotonous eyes with pre-existing choroidal effusions and following penetrating trauma.
2. **Haemorrhage** from the entry site is an uncommon complication which tends to occur at the very beginning of the procedure. The bleeding may be controlled by either increasing the intraocular pressure by elevation of the infusion bottles or by bipolar diathermy.
3. **Incarceration** of vitreous and/or retina into the entry site may occur in eyes with bullous RDs. It can be prevented by plugging the sclerotomies and not starting the intraocular infusion until vitrectomy is about to begin. Any prolapsed vitreous should be abscissed without exerting traction with De Wecker's scissors flush with the surface of the sclera.
4. **Entry-site breaks** may occur immediately behind sclerotomies. It is therefore important to thoroughly examine entry sites at the end of the procedure and treat any breaks appropriately.

Basic vitrectomy

Technique

1. Place a contact lens onto the cornea and remove the scleral plugs.
2. Whilst viewing through the contact lens insert the vitreous cutter and the fibreoptic light pipe through the upper two sclerotomies (Figure 11.1).
3. Excise the central vitreous gel and any associated opacities.
4. Identify and excise the PHF as far anteriorly as possible, usually flush with the posterior border of the vitreous base.

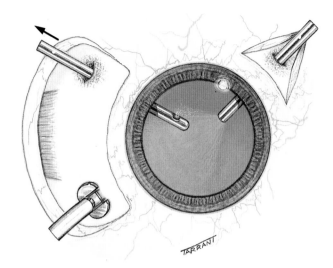

Figure 11.1 Infusion cannula, light pipe and vitreous cutter in position

5. Close the sclerotomies with absorbable sutures and restore the intraocular volume by injection of gas or balanced salt solution.

Potential problems

Miosis

Miosis may occur during periods of hypotony or following inadvertent iris manipulation. To prevent miosis some surgeons advocate a preoperative subconjunctival injection of Mydricaine. Mydriasis may also be restored during surgery either pharmacologically by injecting into the anterior chamber 0.1 ml of a 1:10 000 solution of adrenaline or mechanically by pupil stretching sutures or retractors.

Corneal oedema

1. **Epithelial oedema** is more likely to occur following frequent preoperative instillation of dilating drops and if surgery is unduly prolonged. Visualization of the operating field may be improved by removing the loose epithelium taking care not to damage Bowman's layer and preserving a perilimbal rim of epithelium.
2. **Stromal oedema** with folds in Descemet's membrane occurs more frequently in aphakic eyes and may give rise to annoying distortion and multiple images during fluid-air exchange. Visualization may be improved by coating the endothelial corneal surface with a viscoelastic substance such as Healonid.

149

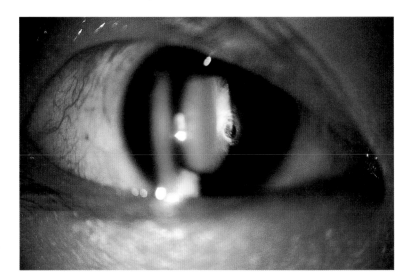

Figure 11.2 Damage to the posterior part of the lens by an instrument during vitrectomy

Lens opacification

Induced lens opacification may result from the following:

1. **Lens touch** by an intraocular instrument is a rare complication (Figure 11.2).
2. **Prolonged surgery**, especially if repeated fluid-gas exchange is required may result in the formation of posterior subcapsular lens opacities.

A lensectomy may have to be performed if lens opacification results in significant impairment of the surgical field which interferes with completion of the procedure.

Haemorrhage

1. **Pre-retinal haemorrhage** may occur during epiretinal membrane dissection especially in the presence of proliferative diabetic retinopathy (see later). The risk of bleeding can be minimized by avoiding traction on neovascular tissue. Small bleeding points can be treated by increasing the intraocular pressure by raising the level of the infusion bottles. Larger bleeders may require treatment with bimanual bipolar diathermy which is attached with clips to the light pipe and backflush needle. The tips of the two instruments are approximated until they almost touch each other at the bleeding point and the diathermy is activated.
2. **Intra-retinal haemorrhage** in attached retina usually follows a forcible avulsion of pre-retinal fibrovascular tissue. The bleeding points can be sealed only with the use of unimanual bipolar diathermy by approximating the tip

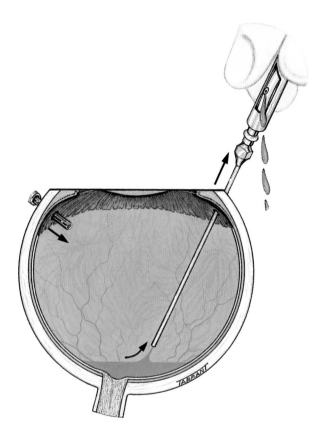

Figure 11.3 Evacuation of blood with a flute needle

of the diathermy to the bleeding point and activating the diathermy directly over it. A fresh haemorrhage leads to the formation of an adherent blood clot which can be peeled from the surface of the retina whereas old residual loose blood can be evacuated with a flute needle (Figure 11.3).

3. **Expulsive suprachoroidal haemorrhage** is a devastating but fortunately very rare complication which is more likely to occur following periods of hypotony, especially in highly myopic aphakic eyes. If recognized early the bleeding may be controlled by the maintenance of a very high intraocular pressure and prompt closure of the entry sites. Drainage of the suprachoroidal blood at the time of surgery is ineffective because clotting occurs immediately. For this reason drainage should be delayed for 10–14 days until the blood clot has lysed.

The above basic steps and potential problems apply to all vitrectomies. Subsequent steps depend on the characteristics of the RD.

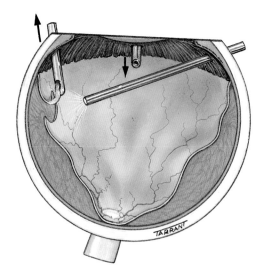

Figure 11.4 Trimming of a flap of a large tear with the cutter

Large or posterior retinal breaks

Vitrectomy

1. If necessary, trim or remove the flap of a large retinal tear (Figure 11.4) as an excessive amount of vitreous in front of the break may interfere with subsequent internal fluid-air exchange.
2. Mark all retinal breaks with bipolar diathermy to cause a localized retinal whitening adjacent to the break. Unless this is carried out it may be very difficult or impossible to identify and treat the breaks once the retina has been flattened.

Fluid-air exchange

1. Place the tip of the flute needle over or inside the break.
2. Simultaneously inject air into the vitreous cavity via the infusion line (Figure 11.5).
3. The pressure of the progressively enlarging air bubble will force the subretinal fluid into the flute needle and out of the eye (hydraulic retinal re-attachment).

Retinopexy

Treat the now flat retinal breaks with either trans-scleral cryotherapy or endolaser photocoagulation using minimal destructive energy. Pre-treatment marking of all breaks with

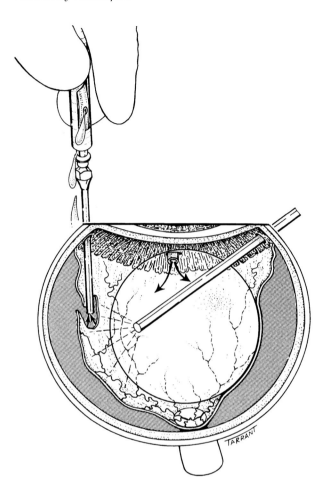

Figure 11.5 Technique of fluid-air exchange

bipolar diathermy is desirable. The merits of scleral buckling in this situation are controversial. There is at least a theoretical rationale of supporting the vitreous base by a narrow encirclement.

Internal tamponade

To achieve prolonged internal tamponade replace the air with a non-expansile concentration of sulphahexafluoride (SF6) or perfluoropropane (C3F8) gases, or with silicone oil. The non-expansile mixture of gas and air is prepared in a large (50 ml) syringe and the air-filled vitreous cavity is flushed with 20% or 30% SF6-air mixture or 14%–16% of C3F8-air mixture.

The technique for treating RD associated with a posterior break is similar. In highly myopic eyes the break may be situated at the edge of a posterior staphyloma or at the macula. In such cases the posterior vitreous may be incompletely detached and it may therefore be difficult to separate the posterior hyaloid from the mobile retina.

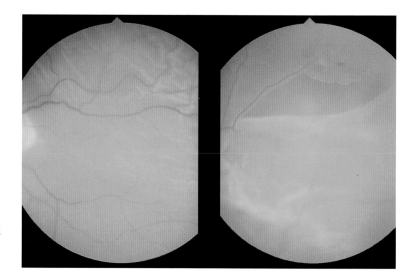

Figure 11.6 Preoperative appearance of a shallow retinal detachment caused by a large posterior tear

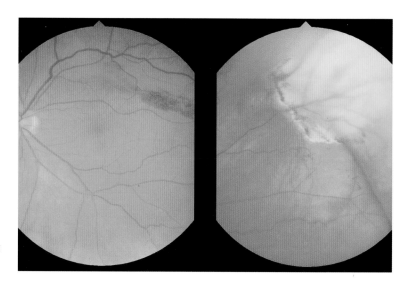

Figure 11.7 Postoperative appearance of the same eye as in the previous figure following successful treatment

Figure 11.6 shows the preoperative appearance of an eye with a shallow RD associated with a large posterior tear and Figure 11.7 shows the postoperative appearance following successful treatment.

Giant retinal tears

Unrolling of flap

Following a complete posterior vitrectomy the flapped over retina is unrolled either bimanually, during a fluid–silicone exchange, or by using 'heavy' perfluorocarbon liquids.

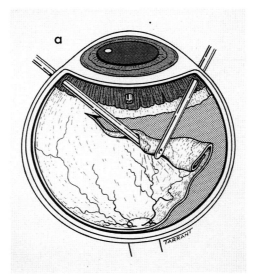

Figure 11.8 Bimanual ('hand-over-hand') technique of unrolling of the flap of a giant retinal tear using the light pipe and vitrectomy probe

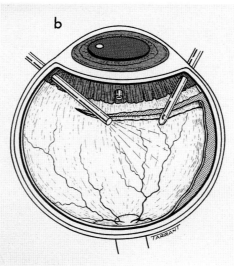

Figure 11.9 Flap of giant tear successfully unrolled

Bimanual technique

1. Using the light pipe in one hand and either a backflush flute needle or vitrectomy probe in the other, gently unroll the everted part of the retina ('hand-over-hand') (Figures 11.8, 11.9).
2. Once the retinal flap is at least partially unrolled, inject silicone through the infusion cannula with the help of either a mechanized injector or a screw syringe (Figure 11.10).
3. Drain the SRF through the tear under direct visualization during silicone-fluid exchange.

Lensectomy and inverting the patient to a prone position during fluid exchange are generally not necessary.

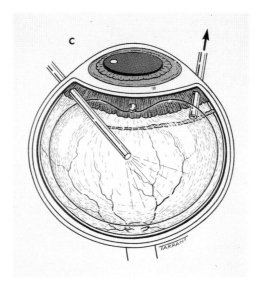

Figure 11.10 Injection of silicone oil after the flap has been unrolled

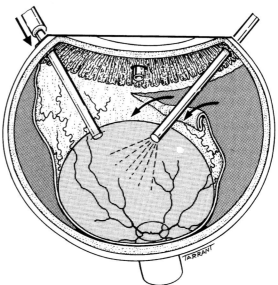

Figure 11.11 Unrolling of flap of a giant tear using heavy liquid

Technique using heavy liquid

1. Under direct visualization slowly inject the heavy liquid over the optic disc.
2. The expanding globule will both unfold the retina and expel the SRF through the giant tear into the vitreous cavity (Figure 11.11) and out of the eye via a flute needle.

Subsequent steps

1. Laser photocoagulation around the tear is performed either directly (i.e. endolaser) or/and via an indirect

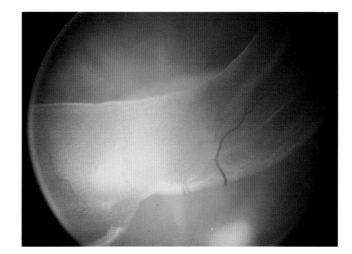

Figure 11.12 Preoperative appearance of retinal detachment caused by a giant tear

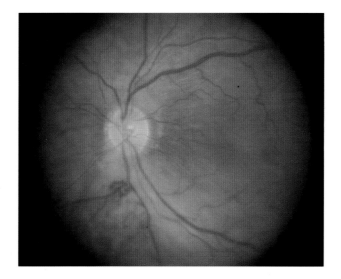

Figure 11.13 Postoperative appearance of same eye as in the previous figure following successful treatment

ophthalmoscope. Laser photocoagulation is preferable to cryotherapy as it is less likely to induce extensive dispersion of the RPE.

2. Scleral buckling is usually not required because most giant tears tend to involve the superior retina and can be closed by internal tamponade. Occasionally, however, the tear may extend below the horizontal meridian and that part of the tear should be supported by a scleral buckle to minimize the risk of re-detachment.

3. Prophylaxis of the fellow eye is mandatory because of the high risk of giant tear formation. Treatment involves either cryotherapy (see Figure 3.12) or the application of two rows of laser photocoagulation to the post-oral retina regardless

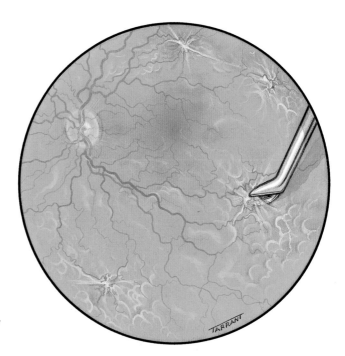

Figure 11.14 Dissection of starfolds in proliferative vitreoretinopathy with vertically cutting scissors

of whether or not vitreoretinal abnormalities such as 'white-without-pressure' are present.

Figure 11.12 shows the preoperative appearance of an RD caused by a giant tear and Figure 11.13 shows the postoperative appearance following successful treatment.

Proliferative vitreoretinopathy

The aims of surgery in PVR are to release transvitreal traction by vitrectomy and tangential (surface) traction by membrane dissection in order to restore retinal mobility and allow closure of retinal breaks.

Membrane dissection

Localised fixed retinal folds ('starfolds') may be freed by the removal of the central plaque of epiretinal membrane as follows:

1. Engage the tip of the vertically cutting scissors in the edge of the valley of the membrane betwen two adjacent retinal folds (Figure 11.14).

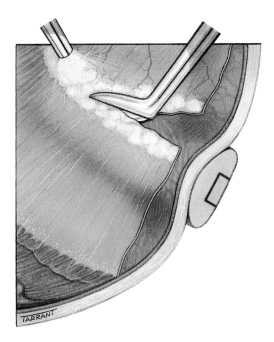

Figure 11.15 Relieving retinotomy in proliferative vitreoretinopathy

2. Pull the membrane towards the ora serrata until it peels from the surface of the retina. If the membrane is too adherent and/or the retina is too mobile transect the membrane with scissors prior to its complete removal. As epiretinal traction is being relieved the retina will become progressively more mobile so that further attempts at membrane dissection may be hampered. The use of heavy liquids to stabilize the posterior retina greatly improves the ability to continue further dissection towards the vitreous base. In the presence of severe contraction of the vitreous base (anterior PVR) it may be necessary to perform a lensectomy in order to complete the dissection.
3. Perform internal fluid-air exchange and apply retinopexy to all retinal breaks.
4. Support the vitreous base by a broad scleral buckle.
5. Exchange the intraocular air for an extended intraocular tamponading agent such as C3F8 or silicone oil.

Relieving retinotomy

The decision to perform a relieving retinotomy is made after epiretinal membrane dissection has been performed as completely as possible but the retinal mobility is deemed insufficient for lasting re-attachment. Because any unrelieved traction tends to be at the vitreous base most retinotomies are sited behind the posterior border of the vitreous base and are

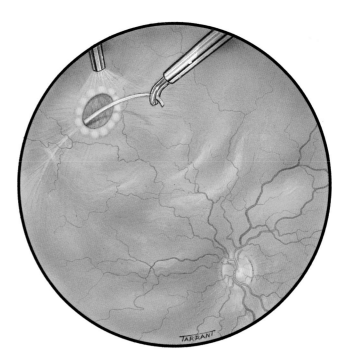

Figure 11.16 Removal of subretinal membrane in proliferative vitreoretinopathy

circumferentially orientated. Occasionally radial retinotomies are used for rigid posterior margins of long-standing retinal tears.

1. Coagulate the retina and its blood vessels using bipolar unimanual or bimanual diathermy with the electrodes attached to the vitreous scissors and to the fibreoptic light pipe.
2. Perform the retinotomy with vertically cutting scissors (Figure 11.15). To be efficient the cut must be large and extend through the inferior 180°.
3. Inject a tamponading agent and drain SRF simultaneously, similar to the technique used to treat giant retinal tears.
4. Excise the anterior flap as far anteriorly as possible and treat the posterior edge of the retinotomy with endolaser photo-coagulation.

Removal of subretinal membranes

Because subretinal membranes are more elastic than those on the retinal surface simply cutting the membrane may be sufficient to release traction.

1. Gain access to the subretinal membrane or band either through a peripheral break or via retinotomy placed directly over the membrane.
2. Remove the cut membrane with forceps (Figure 11.16).

160

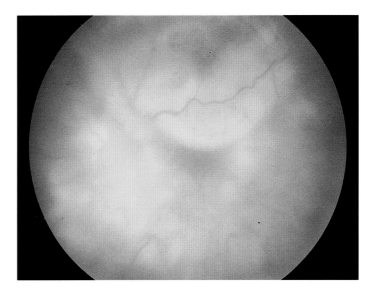

Figure 11.17 Preoperative appearance of an eye with severe proliferative vitreoretinopathy

Figures 11.17, 11.18, 11.19 and 11.20 show the preoperative and postoperative appearances of two eyes with severe proliferative vitreoretinopathy.

Tractional retinal detachment

The goal of vitrectomy in tractional RDs is to release anteroposterior and/or circumferential vitreoretinal traction. Because the membranes are vascularised they cannot be simply peeled from the surface of the retina as in eyes with PVR because this would result in haemorrhage and tearing of the retina. The two methods of removing fibrovascular membranes in diabetic tractional RDs are (a) **delamination** and (b) **segmentation**.

Delamination

Delamination involves the horizontal cutting of the individual vascular pegs connecting the membranes to the surface of the retina. This is preferred to segmentation because it allows the complete removal of fibrovascular tissue from the retinal surface (en-bloc delamination). The technique is as follows:

1. Cut a window in the partially detached posterior hyaloid and pass horizontally cutting scissors into the retrohyaloid space.
2. Gain access to the cleavage between the membrane and the detached retina (Figure 11.21) by elevating a posterior exten-

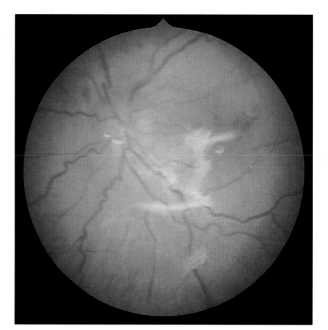

Figure 11.18 Postoperative appearance of same eye as in the previous figure following successful treatment by vitrectomy, membrane peeling and injection of silicone oil

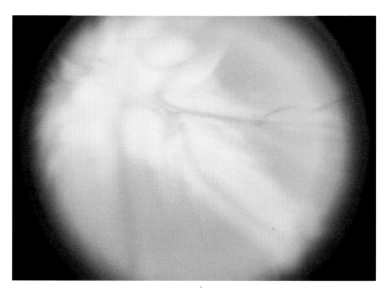

Figure 11.19 Preoperative appearance of an eye with severe proliferative retinopathy

sion of the membrane which is usually adherent to the thin atrophic retina. Failure to find this plane will cause splitting of the membrane leading to haemorrhage and inadequate dissection.

3. Divide the vascular attachments ('pegs') individually as the remaining posterior hyaloid draws the edges of the freed membrane away from the retinal surface. When the membrane has been completely separated the remaining

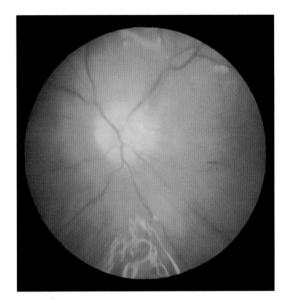

Figure 11.20 Postoperative appearance of same eye as in the previous figure following successful treatment

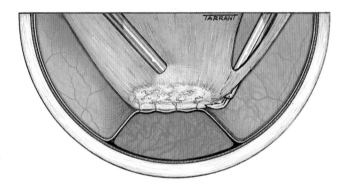

Figure 11.21 Technique of delamination using horizontally cutting scissors

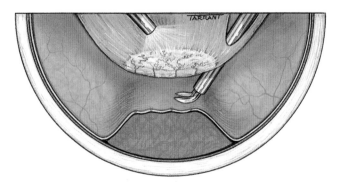

Figure 11.22 Delamination completed

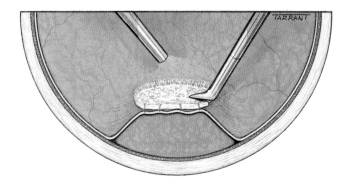

Figure 11.23 Technique of segmentation using vertically cutting scissors

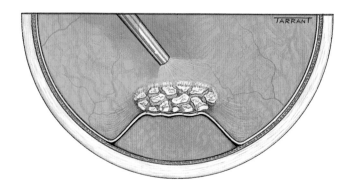

Figure 11.24 Segmentation completed

membrane-posterior hyaloid complex will hang over the retina like a hammock (Figure 11.22).

4. Excise the membrane-posterior hyaloid complex with the cutter.

Segmentation

Segmentation involves the vertical cutting of epiretinal membranes into small segments. It is used to release circumferential vitreoretinal traction when delamination is difficult or impossible, such as in very mobile combined-traction-rhegmatogenous RD associated with posterior retinal breaks. The technique is as follows:

1. Perform a complete vitrectomy and divide the posterior hyaloid attachment to the epiretinal membrane ('truncation' of the posterior hyaloid).
2. Engage the lower blade of vertically cutting scissors in the cleavage space between the membrane and the retinal surface (Figure 11.23).
3. Cut the membrane into small segments usually with the vascular pegs in their centres (Figure 11.24).
4. Seal bleeding points with bipolar diathermy.

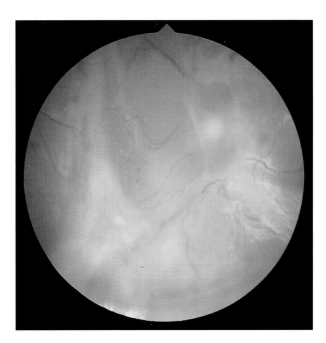

Figure 11.25 Diabetic tractional RD before surgery

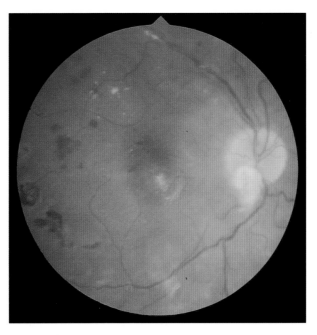

Figure 11.26 Appearance after successful surgery

Provided there are no retinal breaks internal tamponade is not required in the treatment of tractional RDs ('no tear–no air'). However, in the presence of retinal breaks (pre-existing or iatrogenic) hydraulic re-attachment by fluid-air exchange is performed and the edges of the break are treated with

165

retinopexy. In diabetics, internal tamponade with a long-acting gas is preferred to silicone oil. A scleral buckle is usually not required in tractional RDs associated with proliferative diabetic retinopathy, provided iatrogenic breaks associated with entry sites have not been discovered at the completion of surgery.

Figure 11.25 shows the preoperative appearance of a diabetic tractional RD and Figure 11.26 shows the postoperative appearance following successful surgery.

Further reading

Aaberg, T. M. (1988) Management of anterior and posterior proliferative vitreoretinopathy. XLV Edward Jackson Memorial Lecture. *American Journal of Ophthalmology*, **106**, 519–532

Abrams, G. W. (1990) Relaxing retinotomies – analysis of anatomic and visual results. *Ophthalmology*, **97**, 647–648

Blinder, K. J., Peyman, G. A., Paris, C. L. *et al.* (1991) Vitreon, a new perfluorocarbon. *British Journal of Ophthalmology*, **75**, 240–244

Camacho, H., Bajaire, B. and Meija, L. F. (1992) Silicone oil in the management of giant tears. *Annals of Ophthalmology*, **24**, 45–49

Chang, S. (1987) Low viscosity liquid fluorocarbons in vitreous surgery, *American Journal of Ophthalmology*, **103**, 38–43

Chang, S., Lincoff, H. A., Coleman, D. *et al.* (1985) Perfluorocarbon gases in vitreous surgery. *Ophthalmology*, **92**, 651–656

Chang, S., Lincoff, H., Zimmerman, N. J. *et al.* (1989) Giant retinal tears: surgical techniques and results using perfluorocarbon liquids. *Archives of Ophthalmology*, **107**, 761–766

Chang, S., Reppucci, V., Zimmerman, N. J. *et al.* (1989) Perfluorocarbon liquids in the management of traumatic retinal detachment. *Ophthalmology*, **96**, 785–792

Escoffery, R. F., Olk, R. J., Grand, M. G. *et al.* (1985) Vitrectomy without scleral buckling for primary rhegmatogenous retinal detachment. *American Journal of Ophthalmology*, **99**, 275–281

Federman, J. L. and Eagle, R. J. R. (1990) Extensive peripheral retinectomy combined with posterior 360° retinectomy for retinal reattachment in advanced proliferative vitreoretinopathy cases. *Ophthalmology*, **97**, 1305–1320

Glaser, B. M., Carter, J. B., Kupperman, B. D. *et al.* (1991) Perfluorooctane in the treatment of giant retinal tears with proliferative vitreoretinopathy. *Ophthalmology*, **98**, 1613–1621

Gonvers, M. (1985) Temporary silicone oil tamponade in the management of retinal detachment with proliferative vitreoretinopathy. *American Journal of Ophthalmology*, **100**, 239–245

Gremillion, C. M. Jr., Peyman, G. A., Kwan-Rong, L. *et al.* (1990) Fluorosilicone oil in the treatment of retinal detachment. *British Journal of Ophthalmology*, **74**, 643–646

Leaver, P. K., Cooling, R. J., Feretis, E. B. *et al.* (1984) Vitrectomy and fluid/silicone-oil exchange for giant retinal tears. *British Journal of Ophthalmology*, **68**, 432–438

Lopez, R. and Chang, S. (1992) Long-term results of vitrectomy and perfluorocarbons for the treatment of severe vitreoretinopathy. *American Journal of Ophthalmology*, **113**, 424–428

Morse, L. S., McCuen, B. W. II, and Machemer, R. (1990) Relaxing retinotomies: analysis of anatomic and visual results. *Ophthalmology*, **97**, 642–647

Scott, J. (1990) Fluorosilicone oil for retinal detachment. *British Journal of Ophthalmology*, **74,** 614–642

Silicone Study Group. (1992) Vitrectomy with silicone oil or sulphur hexafluoride gas in eyes with severe proliferative vitreoretinopathy: Results of a randomized clinical trial. *Archives of Ophthalmology*, **110,** 770–779

Silicone Study Group. (1992) Vitrectomy with silicone oil or perfluoro-propane gas in eyes with severe proliferative vitreoretinopathy: results of a randomized clinical trial. *Archives of Ophthalmology*, **110,** 780–792

Wilson, H.N. and Leaver, P.K. (1990) Extended criteria for vitrectomy and fluid/silicone oil exchange. *Eye*, **4,** 850–854

12 Postoperative complications of vitrectomy

Raised intraocular pressure

Cataract

Recurrent vitreous haemorrhage

Retinal re-detachment

Raised intraocular pressure

Secondary angle-closure glaucoma

Secondary-angle closure glaucoma may be associated with choroidal swelling and ciliary body rotation. Treatment is with mydriatics and cycloplegics.

Overexpansion of intraocular gas

Raised intraocular pressure may occur as a result of complete filling of the vitreous cavity if the concentration of expansile gas used was inadvertently too high. If the intraocular pressure cannot be controlled medically, 0.5–1 ml of the gas should be removed. This may have to be repeated if the remaining gas continues to expand.

Silicone-associated glaucoma

1. **Early glaucoma** is caused by silicone oil in the anterior chamber (Figure 12.1). This occurs as a result of pupil block, particularly in the aphakic eye with an intact iris diaphragm. The prolonged contact of silicone oil with the corneal endothelium may also give rise to keratopathy (Figure 12.3). In aphakic eyes, both glaucoma and keratopathy can be prevented by performing an inferior iridectomy at the time of the original surgery (Figure 12.4). The iridectomy allows free passage of aqueous to the anterior chamber so that the silicone remains behind the iris plane and does not block the pupil.
2. **Late glaucoma** may occur, probably as a result of trabecular blockage by emulsified silicone in the anterior chamber (Figure 12.2). This complication may be prevented

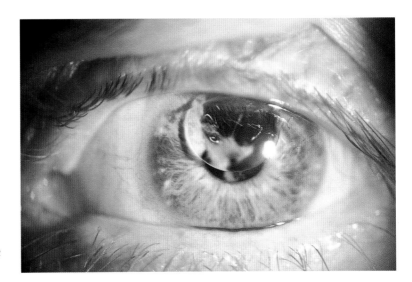

Figure 12.1 Silicone oil in the anterior chamber of an aphakic eye

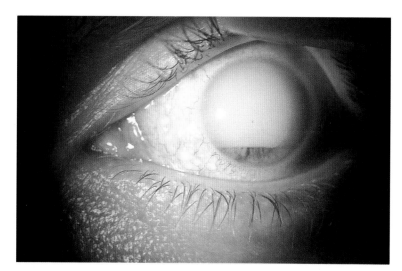

Figure 12.2 Emulsified silicone oil in the anterior chamber

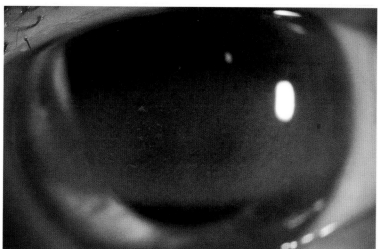

Figure 12.3 Band keratopathy induced by silicone oil

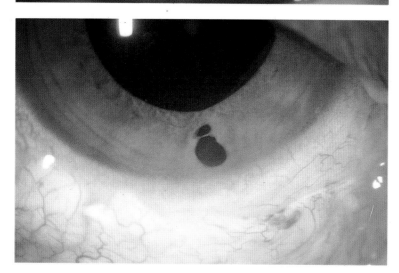

Figure 12.4 Inferior iridectomy in a silicone-filled aphakic eye

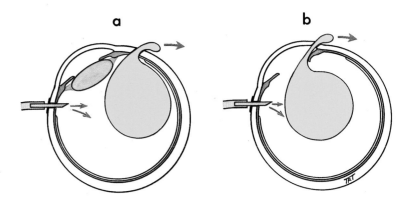

Figure 12.5 Technique of removal of silicone oil. (*a*), In a phakic eye; (*b*), in an aphakic eye

by an early removal of silicone oil either via the pars plana in phakic eyes (Figure 12.5*a*) or the limbus in aphakic eyes (Figure 12.5*b*). Unfortunately, following removal of silicone oil there is a risk of retinal re-detachment (see later).

Ghost cell glaucoma

Following a complete vitrectomy in patients with dense vitreous haemorrhage associated with RD, the residual effete red blood cells may enter the anterior chamber and mechanically block the trabecular meshwork. In most cases medical treatment is sufficient to control the pressure although occasionally an anterior chamber washout may be required.

Steroid-induced glaucoma

The prolonged postoperative use of strong steroids may cause elevation of intraocular pressure in susceptible individuals.

Cataract

Gas-induced

The use of either a large and/or long-lived intravitreal gas bubble almost invariably gives rise to feathering of the posterior subcapsular lens cortex. Fortunately lens opacification is usually transient and can be minimized by using lower concentrations and smaller volumes of gas.

Silicone-induced

Almost all phakic eyes with silicone oil eventually develop cataract. The initial hope that the early removal of silicone would prevent cataract formation has not materialized. If a cataract

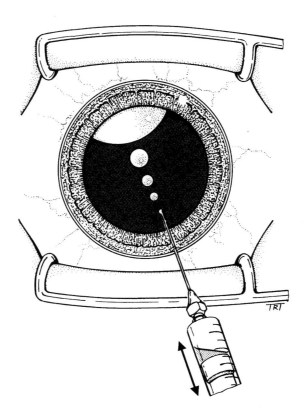

Figure 12.6 Push-pull technique of fluid-gas exchange in treating re-detachment in an aphakic eye

develops, the silicone oil can be removed in conjunction with cataract extraction and posterior chamber lens implantation.

Delayed cataract formation

Following successful vitrectomy a large proportion of eyes develop nuclear sclerosis within 5–10 years.

Recurrent vitreous haemorrhage

Most diabetic eyes develop a transient vitreous haemorrhage within the first two postoperative days following extensive dissection of fibrovascular tissue. If the haemorrhage becomes recurrent or if it persists beyond 3-4 months neovascularization of the anterior hyaloid should be suspected.

Retinal re-detachment

Whilst the initial success rate for retinal re-attachment is generally high, the complex nature of cases requiring vitrectomy puts

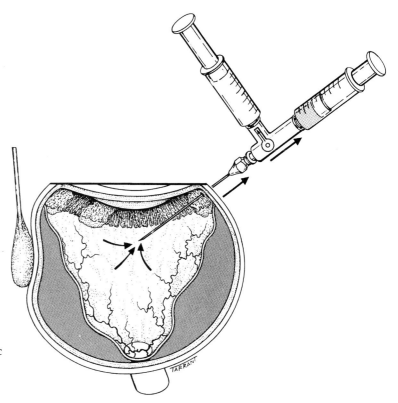

Figure 12.7 First stage of consecutive fluid-gas exchange to treat re-detachment in phakic or pseudophakic eyes showing aspiration of fluid from the vitreous cavity

such eyes at a higher risk of re-detachment. The commonest time for this to occur is when the intraocular gas bubble has absorbed (usually 3-6 weeks postoperatively) or after the removal of silicone oil.

Causes

1. Re-opening of the original break may occur because of either inadequate dissection at the time of original surgery in eyes with PVR or the re-proliferation of epiretinal membranes which is more common in eyes with proliferative diabetic retinopathy.
2. There may be new or missed breaks especially those related to the original pars plana entry sites.
3. Early removal of silicone oil is associated with a 25% risk of retinal re-detachment in eyes with PVR and giant tears, and 11% risk in eyes with proliferative diabetic retinopathy.

Treatment

Because a previously vitrectomized eye has a fluid-filled vitreous cavity further fluid-gas exchange can be performed with relative ease under local anaesthesia. In aphakic eyes this can be

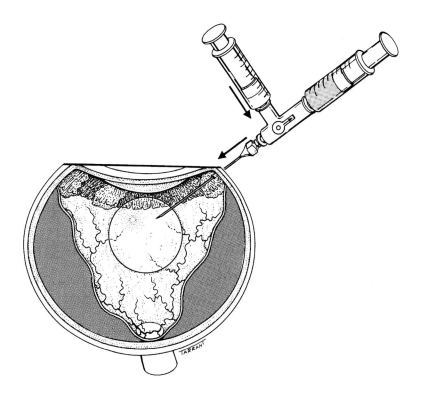

Figure 12.8 Second stage of fluid-gas exchange showing injection of gas

done at the slitlamp through the limbus by a 'push-pull' technique (Figure 12.6). In phakic or pseudo-phakic eyes fluid-gas exchange can be performed through the pars plana with the patient lying down (Figures 12.7, 12.8). Following further face-down positioning the retina usually re-attaches and the breaks can be treated by laser photocoagulation using the indirect ophthalmoscopic delivery system.

Further reading

Ando, F. (1985) Intraocular hypertension resulting from pupillary block by silicone oil. *American Journal of Ophthalmology*, **99**, 87–88

Beekhuis, W. H., Ando, F. and Zivojnovic, R. (1985) Silicone oil keratopathy: Indications for keratoplasty. *British Journal of Ophthalmology*, **69**, 247–253

Beekhuis, W. H., Ando, F., Zivojnovic, R. *et al.* (1987) Basal iridectomy at 6 o'clock in the aphakic eye treated with silicone oil: prevention of keratopathy and secondary glaucoma. *British Journal of Ophthalmology*, **71**, 197–200

Casswell, A. G. and Gregor, Z. J. (1987) Silicone oil removal. I. The effect on the complications of silicone oil. *British Journal of Ophthalmology*, **71**, 893–897

Casswell, A. G. and Gregor, Z. J. (1987) Silicone oil removal.II. Operative and postoperative complications. *British Journal of Ophthalmology*, **71,** 898–902

Federman, J. L. and Schubert, H. D. (1988) Complications associated with the use of silicone oil in 150 eyes after retina-vitreous surgery. *Ophthalmology*, **95,** 870–876

Kampik, A., Hoing, C., Heidenkummer, H-P. (1992) Problems and timing of removal of silicone oil. *Retina*, **12,** s11–s16

Lewis, H. and Aaberg, T. M. (1991) Causes of failure after repeated vitreoretinal surgery for recurrent vitreoretinopathy. *American Journal of Ophthalmology*, **111,** 15–19

Lewis, H., Aaberg, T. M. and Abrams, G. W. (1991) Causes of failure after initial vitreoretinal surgery for severe proliferative vitreoretinopathy. *American Journal of Ophthalmology*, **111,** 8–14

Index

Note: Numbers in **bold** refer to pages on which illustrations appear.